Urban Action Networks

Urban Action Networks

HIV/AIDS and Community Organizing in New York City

Howard Lune

ROWMAN & LITTLEFIELD PUBLISHERS, INC.
Lanham • Boulder • New York • Toronto • Plymouth, UK

ROWMAN & LITTLEFIELD PUBLISHERS, INC.

Published in the United States of America
by Rowman & Littlefield Publishers, Inc.
A wholly owned subsidiary of The Rowman & Littlefield Publishing Group, Inc.
4501 Forbes Boulevard, Suite 200, Lanham, Maryland 20706
www.rowmanlittlefield.com

Estover Road, Plymouth PL6 7PY, United Kingdom

Portions of chapters 1, 5, and 7 were published earlier as "Embedded Systems: The Case
of HIV/AIDS Nonprofit Organizations in New York City," Howard Lune and Hillary
Oberstein, 2001, *Voluntas: International Journal of Voluntary and Nonprofit
Organizations* 12, no. 1. With kind permission of Springer Science and Business Media.

Portions of chapter 4 were published as "Weathering the Storm: Nonprofit Organization
Survival Strategies in a Hostile Climate," *Nonprofit and Voluntary Sector Quarterly* 31,
no. 4, December 2002.

British Library Cataloguing in Publication Information Available

Library of Congress Cataloging-in-Publication Data

Lune, Howard, 1962–
   Urban action networks : HIV/AIDS and community organizing in New York City /
Howard Lune.
      p. cm.
   Includes bibliographical references and index.
   ISBN-13: 978-0-7425-4083-5 (cloth : alk. paper)
   ISBN-10: 0-7425-4083-9 (cloth : alk. paper)
   ISBN-13: 978-0-7425-4084-2 (pbk. : alk. paper)
   ISBN-10: 0-7425-4084-7 (pbk. : alk. paper)
   1. AIDS (Disease)—New York (State)—New York. 2. AIDS (Disease)—Social
aspects—New York (State)—New York. 3. AIDS (Disease)—Patients—Services for—
New York (State)—New York. 4. Community health services—New York (State)—
New York. I. Title.
RA643.84.N7L86 2007
362.196'97920097471—dc22

                                                                                    2006027005

Printed in the United States of America

⊗™ The paper used in this publication meets the minimum requirements of American
National Standard for Information Sciences—Permanence of Paper for Printed Library
Materials, ANSI/NISO Z39.48-1992.

Contents

Contents

Abbreviations

COMMUNITY-BASED ORGANIZATIONS

ACT UP	AIDS Coalition to Unleash Power
ACQC	AIDS Center of Queens County
ACRIA	AIDS Community Research Initiative of America
ADAPT	Association for Drug Abuse Prevention and Treatment
AmFAR	American Foundation for AIDS Research
APICHA	Asian and Pacific Islander Coalition on HIV/AIDS
APLA	AIDS Project Los Angeles
ARC	AIDS Resource Center/Bailey House
ASC	AIDS Service Center of Lower Manhattan
BATF	Brooklyn AIDS Task Force
BP	Body Positive
BC/EFA	Broadway Cares/Equity Fights AIDS
CHP	Community Health Project, now Callen-Lorde Community Health Center
DAAIR	Direct AIDS Alternative Information Resources
DIFFA	The Design Industry Foundation for AIDS
FID	Friends in Deed
FROST'D	Foundation for Research on Sexually Transmitted Diseases
GLAAD	Gay and Lesbian Alliance against Defamation
GLWD	God's Love We Deliver
GMAD	Gay Men of African Descent
GMHC	Gay Men's Health Crisis
HAF	Hispanic AIDS Forum

HCA	Haitian Coalition on AIDS
HCC	Haitian Centers Council
HEAL	Health Education AIDS Liaison
LCOA	Latino Commission on AIDS
MDHG	Amsterdam's Interest Group for Drug Users
MTFA	Minority Task Force on AIDS
MV	Mothers' Voices
NAB	National AIDS Brigade
NYHRE	New York Harm Reduction Educators
PHP	Positive Health Project
PWAC	People with AIDS Coalition
PWA HG	People with AIDS Health Group
SACHR	St. Ann's Corner of Harm Reduction
TAG	Treatment Action Group
T+D	ACT UP Treatment and Data Committee
WARN	Women and AIDS Resource Network

AGENCIES AND TECHNICAL TERMS

ACTG	AIDS Clinical Trials Group
AHSP	AIDS Health Services Program
AIDS	Acquired Immune Deficiency Syndrome
AI	AIDS Institute
ASO	AIDS service organization
ATEU	AIDS Treatment and Evaluation Unit
AZT	Azidothymidine
CARE Act	Ryan White Comprehensive AIDS Emergency Resources Act
CBO	community-based organizations
CCWG	Community Constituency Working Group
CDC	Centers for Disease Control and Prevention
CSP	Community Service Program
DOH	Department of Health
DAS	NYC Division of AIDS Services
ESAP	Expanded Syringe Access Program
FDA	Food and Drug Administration
GRID	Gay Related Immune Deficiency
HIV	Human Immunodeficiency Virus
HRSA	Health Resources and Services Administration
HUD	Housing and Urban Development

IDU	injecting drug user
KS	Kaposi's Sarcoma
NEP	needle exchange programs
NIAID	National Institute on Allergies and Infectious Diseases
NIH	National Institutes of Health
NPO	nonprofit organization
OAR	Office of AIDS Research
ONDCP	The White House Office of National Drug Control Policy
PCP	*Pneumocystis* pneumonia
PLWHIV/AIDS	people living with HIV/AIDS
PWA	People with AIDS
RFP	request for proposal
RWJF	Robert Wood Johnson Foundation
SEP	syringe exchange programs

Introduction:
Boundaries and Borders

In March 1994, I marched across the Brooklyn Bridge toward New York's City Hall with about five hundred other people. There was a great deal of diversity in the group, by age, gender, ethnicity, style of dress, and so on. As the exit ramp in downtown Manhattan came into view, the group of mostly youngish men around me were loudly chanting: "Hey Hey, Ho Ho, Julie Andrews has got the glow!" Why they were doing this is a very complex matter, and the desire to explain it is one of the principle motivations underlying this book.

The event marked the kickoff of the "Target Rudy" campaign, and the target was, indeed, New York City's new mayor, Rudolph Giuliani, who had recently taken office. Giuliani was a Republican in a traditionally Democratic city, and he had risen to power on a "tough on crime" platform that had a lot to say about individual responsibility, much less to say about government responsibility, and hardly a word about HIV/AIDS. The community was worried. Then, on Friday, March 18, late in the day for a news announcement, the mayor offered his first significant position statement on the topic. He suggested that the city's Division of AIDS Services (DAS), the largest service organization for people living with HIV/AIDS in the city, in which an estimated thirteen thousand were in need of such services (U.S. Department of Health and Human Services 1995), was not necessary. He suggested that he might shut it down.

So, why were we on the bridge chanting odd slogans? First, we were there because the new mayor had issued a challenge to "the AIDS community," an ambiguously defined, rapidly shifting, politically inconsistent, angry, conciliatory, powerful, disenfranchised network of private individuals and nonprofit organizations (NPOs) that had risen to remarkable prominence on the wave of the emergence of the AIDS Coalition to Unleash Power (ACT UP) in 1987, only to devolve into something more scattered and controllable in the early 1990s. Mayor Giuliani, who, the city would quickly learn, did not like to be pressured by outsiders, wanted to see if there was any fight left in the community.

We were there because the community wanted to show that it could still fight. The date and time, only one full workday after the mayor's provocative announcement, were chosen in part to demonstrate that the activist phone tree still worked and that a lot of people from a lot of organizations could be mobilized on short notice. In fact, many of the marchers had been anxiously awaiting just such a threat, or opportunity. The generally promising tone of the previous administration under David Dinkins and the recent influx of federal money through the Ryan White Comprehensive AIDS Resources Emergency (CARE) Act had led many in the HIV/AIDS field to let the government take the lead in policy and services, at least locally, and to try not to make too many waves. Many of the activists felt stifled and undermined, and some admitted to being almost glad to have an openly hostile mayor against whom they could actually generate some public actions. The two extremes were testing one another.

We were there because there was an interorganizational network of great complexity and depth running through the community, or at least through the organized parts of it. Years of coordinated activity, formal and informal exchanges, self-reliance, fund-raising, consciousness raising, self-help, self-recriminations, and all sorts of personal mobility and interpersonal linkages throughout this field of action had created a dense web of communications and mobilization potential. ACT UP/NY—the AIDS Coalition to Unleash Power—had taken the lead on making the calls and designing the "March as if your life depended on it" flyer. Stand Up Harlem had written many of the announcements and printed statements, though GMHC—Gay Men's Health Crisis—was one of the few groups that could afford to provide all of the necessary photocopying and faxing. Mothers' Voices (MV) brought out their unique community of support, primarily professional women with HIV-positive family members, while God's Love We Deliver (GLWD) brought out their volunteer base, many of whom were young and underemployed.

I was there because I was trying to study this very network. I was at that place at that time because I had been conducting interviews at ACT UP/NY during the past month, and so I had become connected to the activist alert system. I marched up toward the front with those contacts where I could observe more, not yet recognizing how the order of the march had been determined. ACT UP, the hardest core of street activists in the community, went first so that they would be the ones arrested when we reached the police cordon.

Stand Up Harlem, ADAPT (Alcohol and Other Drug Abuse Prevention Team), and other organizations representing the interests of drug users and former users moved further back to avoid arrest. Many of their people were still on parole or probation from drug-related convictions. Another arrest, even for disturbing the peace, would violate the terms of their release and trigger the resumption of a potentially lengthy prison sentence. I would learn all of this very soon, as we reached a point far enough onto the bridge to be invisible from either shore and were met by the largest single gathering of police I had ever seen. In an orderly and peaceful fashion, as though rehearsed many times before, the police opened the doors to their paddy wagons while the ACT UP group moved defiantly, but unthreateningly, past the "line in the sand" and sat down. I moved back to join the Harlem group and to await police instructions regarding when and where we would be allowed to continue.

The whys of the situation were as complex as the network itself. Chanting slogans is a standard part of the repertoire of contentious politics, and we had run through many of them as we walked. Though the marchers had come together under so many organizational banners to show solidarity against the city (in support of a city agency), they were not of a single voice. The DAS worked closely with most of the community's privately organized service agencies and even shared key funding sources with them. Thus, many of the groups represented on the bridge had made the transition from outsiders to insiders in the domain of health policy and HIV/AIDS service delivery. Others aggressively opposed the professionalization of the community and reveled in their amateur status. ACT UP exemplified this position and drew as well upon the lesbian and gay activist community's history of camp and showmanship. In their hands, the staidly predictable phrase "Giuliani has got to go" wound its way through a wave of spontaneous variants before settling for a time on the incongruous Julie Andrews reference.

The ability of so many diverse groups and voices to act in concert was one of the few remaining factors that made the organized HIV/AIDS community a community at all. Their ability to coordinate was a strength, as was their ability to remain diverse. Negotiating between these two needs might have been the most difficult conceptual challenge to the community, and it made for odd identity politics. To their advantage, the government did not know how to get a fix on the HIV/AIDS community, and so they could still surprise and upset their targets. To their annoyance, the media did not understand them either, and showed little interest in doing so. On the Manhattan side of the bridge, organizers had set up information booths with press kits and appointed representatives, anxious to explain the day's events. Very few of them were seen on television or quoted in the press. On the other hand, the most flamboyant supporters, including men in drag who raced by on inline skates, delighted the cameras. When questioned by reporters, their inability to succinctly explain what the DAS did or why it had to be saved made some of the news stories that much more amusing. Such distractions watered down the rally's potential effectiveness, and some participants wondered if they could impose a dress code on a public protest.

This conflict also exemplified one of the strengths of the organized community's decentralized form. HIV/AIDS brought together a wide assortment of socially marginalized groups including gay men, injecting drug users, uninsured minority families, and women in sexually exploitive relationships. None of them had had much say in politics before HIV/AIDS, and their collective association with the plague of the twentieth century did not empower them. In such circles, democratic participation was highly valued, and no form of censorship was likely to find support. However frustrating it might be to the official spokespersons, the community needed to show that every voice counted and that all participants were wanted. This was what made them different from the government agencies with or against whom they worked.

STATE AND COMMUNITY

The community-based mobilization of affected peoples in response to HIV/ AIDS has been remarkable and nearly unprecedented. Activists, advocates, and community-based organizations (CBOs) have laid their imprint on all facets of our understanding of HIV/AIDS, our responses to it, and the prospects for a future resolution. "What do CBOs do?" Dennis Altman asked in his 1994 study *Power and Community.* "The obvious retort to the question . . . is, of course, 'Everything': there is virtually no aspect of HIV-related work in which there is not involvement by one community group or another" (Altman 1994, 37). His observation echoed numerous other studies of community work. The Philadelphia Commission on AIDS's *Report to the Community* noted that, "for the first seven years of the AIDS epidemic," CBOs provided "virtually all human services for persons with AIDS in Philadelphia" (quoted in Perrow and Guillén 1990, 74). Michael Quam and Nancy Ford, looking at the nationwide mobilization against AIDS, came to the same conclusion. "What have these organizations actually done? One is tempted to answer, everything. They have been the principal and in many locales the only purveyors of clear, explicit, and culturally appropriate education for risk reduction, especially among the gay population" (1990, 42). Ron Bayer and David Kirp contrasted community-based efforts with state-centered ones: "Throughout the epidemic's early years, the volunteer efforts of gay community-based groups provided an extraordinary array of social services to those with HIV-related disease. Such efforts had met needs where government had failed" (Bayer and Kirp 1992, 42).

The contrast between state and community in the response to HIV/AIDS lies at the heart of most of the significant events in the history of AIDS in the United States. Peter Arno and Karyn Feiden, in their study of the development of community involvement in clinical trials, were more explicit about this distinction. Whereas community activists demonstrated extraordinary courage and conviction, "the absence of forceful direction at the highest levels of government has been nothing less than criminal—and it remains so" (1992, 4). The accomplishments of the community groups during the first ten years of the epidemic are all the more remarkable due to their marginality, their outsider status. The relative lack of public-sector accomplishments over the same period is remarkable for analogous reasons. The various agencies of local and federal government and the public health sector are the very institutions from which the community organizations were marginalized. This contrast between the public- and private-sector responses both reflects and reproduces the tensions between the center and the periphery, the world as we try to make it and the world as it is. Yet the relationship is far more complex than the dichotomies described by many writers, particularly those writing in the first decade, fueled by anger and disillusion, for the accomplishments of the community-based collective actors are primarily reflected in the degree to which public policies and programs have come to incorporate their initiatives and personnel.

The conflict between public and private agencies, between state and civil society, in the response to HIV/AIDS has been elaborated many times (Altman 1988; Cain 1995; Padgug 1987; Shilts 1987; Wolfe 1994). The standard format of this narrative relies on the contrast between private, usually gay, male heroes and indifferent, or cowardly, bureaucratic villains. This work will not attempt to reiterate (or contradict) that case. My interest lies with the organizational activities of those activists and advocates who made up the grassroots response, with their organizational accomplishments rather than their social or medical ones. The focus of this study is on uncovering the mobilization processes of new nonprofit organizations started by members of the affected communities, with reference to the institutional environments in which they were embedded. I attempt to follow these groups from their neighborhoods to the urban level and on to the national level or beyond. To the extent that it is possible to recreate a recent history, I begin with the origins of the field and the founding of the first organizations and follow the trajectory of community organizing from outside the domain of public health policy to inside. One important question for this study, then, is How did they get here from there?

The answer to that question cannot be found in the history of any single organization. Rather, the specific accomplishment was in the creation of a new organizational field. This field, which encompasses social movement organizations, service agencies, support groups, treatment research organizations, and a host of other nonprofits, also expanded to incorporate government agencies from health care to law enforcement. It depended on the participation of private-sector pharmaceutical research firms and other companies associated with the public health field, companies that are used to working with the state but had no significant prior experience with community-based mobilizations. In its depth and complexity, the HIV/AIDS field may be compared with many other policy arenas in which the public good is discussed. The seemingly unique feature of this field is that it was generated by community-based nonprofits who then pressed their priorities onto state agencies. Although there is not a great deal of research on the origins of organizational fields, the literature on citizen participation in policy debates often depicts the organized communities as responding to opportunities and threats that originate in government circles rather than as creating these opportunities. Clearly, both occur.

The relationship between members of the organized HIV/AIDS community and government agencies is complex and fluid, as the Target Rudy event demonstrated. Collectively, the community-based groups have worked both with and against the state, sometimes supporting one state agency against another. It is helpful to consider the organized community in contrast to the polity, which we may view as the full range of state-centered social institutions, centered on the government but extending deeply into all aspects of public life (Jepperson 1991), including those private organizations that routinely interact with the state in its own domain (Tilly 1978). While responsibility and authority for HIV/AIDS policies lies with the administrative arms of state and federal government, implementation of such policies often falls to relatively independent social actors, many of whom share the community's priorities. Thus, visible attacks by community groups on policy makers were often balanced by quiet alliances between these groups and members of the public health and law enforcement sectors. It is, I believe, the diversity of these efforts, coupled with the community's ability to define a collective identity, that allowed them to construct a coordinated field of work without central authority. In a similar vein, it was the state's inability to do the same that gave the organized community so much influence over the development of all HIV/AIDS-related work in the United States.

STATE AND CITY

The first reports on what would become known as HIV/AIDS identified fifteen inexplicable cases of *Pneumocystis* pneumonia (PCP) and twenty-six of Kaposi's Sarcoma (KS) among relatively young men in Los Angeles and New York City (Centers for Disease Control [CDC] 1981a, 1981b). From that day to the present, New York has been the epicenter for AIDS in the United States. As of December 2000, New York City reported the highest AIDS case load of any metropolitan area, with more incidents than the next four areas combined (CDC 2000). San Francisco had comparable rates per population size, but with many fewer people and a very different pattern of urban politics and public health.

HIV/AIDS incidence rates in New York City followed the patterns of both the wealthiest and the poorest nations. For those who could afford it, the city offered some of the best health care options in the world, including a high concentration of HIV expertise. For the rest, the city could boast of having more people with virtually no health care at all than many cities have residents. As of 2000, over 1.5 million New Yorkers received Medicaid, and the Division of AIDS Services (DAS), which provides case management and limited medical insurance for low-income people with AIDS, had more than twenty-eight thousand clients (HRA 2000). Neither of these services reaches the majority of homeless New Yorkers, whose numbers have not been consistently estimated.

Ordinarily, the worlds of the haves and have-nots do not visibly intersect. In certain arenas, however, citizens of the two New Yorks may coexist. Ethnic diversity crosses class lines and provides personal, political, and cultural links among people from different social strata. Political activism, which has a long tradition in New York, also brings together otherwise surprising fellow travelers. Collective action and visible community leaders have brought relatively disenfranchised neighborhoods and groups into urban policy arenas and electoral politics (Abu-Lughod 1994). And the material resources and expertise in New York sometimes also "trickle down" in the form of investment in services and infrastructure. Top-rated public hospitals and public clinics share health expertise with all those who need it. Community-development investment provides space, technology, and expertise for nonprofit organizing. Even the homeless in New York City had their own newspaper, *Streetnews*, with a wide readership throughout the 1980s.

The environment for HIV/AIDS in New York was also relatively unique for demographic reasons. The city hosts a large, relatively open, relatively politicized gay community and a large, but mostly hidden, population of injecting drug users. The size of the two most vulnerable population categories in the early years of HIV/AIDS provided conditions for the rapid spread of the virus. The density of the social worlds allowed the condition to reach epidemic proportions prior to any significant anti-AIDS mobilization; exposure to HIV spread far more quickly than relevant prevention information. Yet the size and density of the most affected social groups also provided the conditions for an organized response—social networks with active channels for rapid communication, access to resources, activist histories, and a sense of collective social identity that occasionally included an explicit awareness of collective interests. New York City was therefore both the nation's epicenter for HIV/AIDS and the center of collective organizing in its wake.

CITY AND COMMUNITY

No reliable data exist on the exact number of HIV/AIDS-related community-based organizations operating at any given time, but various estimates and self-reports suggest that as many as two hundred to three hundred organizations may have been in existence in and around New York City in the early 1990s. As of the third quarter of 1997, for example, the CDC National AIDS Clearinghouse listed 261 organizations in New York City, out of a database containing three thousand local and national community-based nonprofit organizations throughout the country. By 1994, according to Johannes Van Vugt, "over 650 community-based organizations, receiving a mix of private, public, and individual funding, [were] registered with, or members of, the National AIDS Network" (1994, 3). The oldest CBOs date back to the earliest appearances of HIV/AIDS in 1981. The configuration of the early field of work was determined primarily by interactions among lesbian and gay community groups attempting to establish their own mandate in the absence of a clear state agenda, but the network of the early 1990s was vastly more diverse and intricately interwoven.

Community-based AIDS work in New York City grew out of existing organizational structures mostly within the politicized gay community (itself not a singular entity). One informant to this work, an activist from the earliest days of HIV, described the gay community as the "building block" of AIDS work to which others looked for leadership. As others recognized HIV/AIDS in their communities, "The Black and Latino communities . . . learned from the gay community." This base of community mobilizing provided a communal identity, a communications network, access to resources, and significant activist experience with which others could align themselves (Elbaz 1992; Epstein 1996). The newly emergent, loosely organized associations, mostly in and around the neighborhood of Chelsea, gave rise to, and ultimately dominated, one of the largest and most rapidly established community-based mobilizations in U.S. history.

The post-Stonewall gay community in New York had been active in political, social, and health issues, but it was relatively quiescent just prior to the onset of HIV/AIDS. One activist in the present study called this mobilization base a "social network with no purpose" on which the "incredible success of [early] AIDS work" relied. Yet the popular association between "gay" and

"AIDS" undermined the improved social standing of lesbians and gays in New York (Siegel, Lune, and Meyer 1998). As many gay rights activists were loath to take on a new source of social stigma (Kowalewski 1988), AIDS-oriented gay organizers quickly differentiated their work as a separate sphere of activity. AIDS itself became the focal point for a new alliance of rights activists, patient advocates, researchers, clinicians, educators, and writers.

Established private organizations that predated HIV/AIDS showed similar reluctance to adapt to its appearance. In her extensive study of the organizational infrastructure of health care in New York, Melinda Cuthbert identified a consistent unwillingness on the part of drug treatment centers, home care agencies, and other preexisting health and service CBOs to add AIDS care to their missions. "Informants from all sectors indicated that most of the traditional voluntary organizations kept a low profile and just avoided responding" (1990, 58). To service providers with narrowly defined missions, HIV/AIDS was too new and too far afield to simply absorb into existing practices. With neither government support nor the resources of the health care field, the new HIV/AIDS CBOs defined and populated the organizational field of HIV/AIDS work in the city.

COMMUNITY AND ORGANIZATION

Like most infectious diseases, HIV/AIDS first appeared as a condition of outcasts (Fee and Fox 1988). Like most comparable afflictions, it can affect anyone, without regard for their social standing. But, having been so afflicted, the infected persons discover that they have been cast out, thus reaffirming the initial stereotype (Sontag 1989). The affected people who organized against HIV/AIDS—those who challenged the stigmas, provided care for the sick, supported treatment research, or conducted the research—necessarily operated from the margins and organized as a collective representation of the peripheral, the deviant, and the unwanted.

For those who were already disdained, for whatever reason, such collective action often provided a sense of empowerment (Siegel, Lune, and Meyer 1998). For the many established medical professionals, political leaders, and others of "good standing," the stigmas attached to HIV/AIDS could be contagious. Those who showed too much empathy could be discredited by association. Entering into AIDS work in the early 1980s amounted to a career-altering decision from which there could be no reasonable expectation of return (Galatowitch 1996).

Despite the lack of help from institutional and other external sources, the new HIV/AIDS organizations undertook high-risk and/or low-reward work in areas that had not been predefined. Motivations internal to the communities have included the sense that "if we don't, who will?" as many informants have suggested, or more simply, the awareness of a need. Disease demographics contributed significantly to the growth of the field as high incidence rates within a population group made it imperative for that group to respond. Many organizers refer to the "threshold" point, at which too many people in one's circles have been "struck down," leading them to take action. When a significant number of people within a population group mobilize around an issue within that community and on behalf of that community, organizational actors refer to that as "owning the issue" (Schneider 1997). For many, it was precisely the perception that the public health institutions were not responding appropriately to HIV/AIDS that led them and their communities to take ownership of their own collective illness experiences (Stoller 1995). The earliest AIDS-related community mobilizations were therefore perceived as substitutes or stopgap measures in the absence of a government-centered response.

The communities of people affected by HIV/AIDS may be collectively identified by the presence of HIV/AIDS in their lives. Yet, beyond the fact of their common exclusion from the institutions on which their lives depended, they were in no way united as a single group or community. Technically, there are no criteria for establishing the boundaries of a community, counting its members, or even knowing whether you yourself are a part of one. On the other hand, a community is real if the people in it see themselves as such. Yet, as Iris Young observed, "in the United States today, identification as a member of such a community also often occurs as an oppositional differentiation from other groups, who are feared or at best devalued" (1990, 311). In this case, the community in question was an unplanned collection of people most often excluded from, and devalued by, conventional notions of American communities. Writers inside and outside of the affected communities used the shorthand "AIDS community" to refer to the collective interests and actions of the affected people, but it was at best a convenient misnomer. To the extent that it occurred, their ability to act as a community of interest or to view themselves as part of a single, broadly defined population was an accomplishment. It was the outcome, not the cause of their collective organizing. It is, in essence, the thing to be explained.

THE INTERORGANIZATIONAL
NETWORK AS A COMMUNITY

Exploratory work on the nonprofit sector as a whole has suggested that interorganizational linkages, both within and beyond the sector, serve to coordinate efforts and manage uncertainty in much the same way that formal structures and contracts do in the for-profit sector (Blau and Rabenovic 1991). Whereas commercial activities occur within specific industries, the context for nonprofit activities is somewhat broader. Call this context the "field" of work. This study examines the emergence and growth of the field of community-based nonprofit groups engaged in HIV/AIDS-related work in New York City. I will refer to this collective as the organized AIDS community. The rest of the HIV/AIDS organizational field—the numerous state agencies; individual social actors; and private, for-profit organizations, including pharmaceutical corporations—only appear in this story to the extent that they interact with the organized AIDS community. For the most part, I will be discussing the organizational identities and missions of the members of this field. To understand organizational identities in the context of an organizational field, we need to look at the various links among the participating groups, where they came from, and what conditions enabled or constrained relations among organizations in this community.

As the organized AIDS community grew and changed, their relations with agencies of the state also shifted. A great deal of the organizing that occurred at the community level may be read as attempts to influence the relations between the state and the community. For the most part, the two sectors competed for influence, as the community sought inroads into the state sector while resisting co-optation for as long as possible. Ultimately the state "won," defining a system of HIV/AIDS research, services, and care that incorporated community groups in a state-centered model. Yet, given the state's reluctance to participate at all in these issues and the disdain for community organizations expressed at the highest levels of government, this new state-community partnership must be considered a measure of the community's success. Furthermore, as this analysis will show, the state-centered model that came to dominate in the early to mid-1990s was, for the most part, created by community groups and adopted by the state.

With each shift in the collective identity, or image, of the HIV/AIDS community, there was a corresponding shift in the configuration of state-community relations. When members of the organized community referred to themselves as "outsiders," it was the polity from which they were excluded. When they speak of "insider tactics," it is with reference to work within the polity. If the organized community consciously organized as a community rather than as a set of independent though interacting groups, then one of the key shared interests within this community was the desire to gain influence within the state-centered policy domains that affected them. I therefore suggest that the dynamic system of interorganizational relations that characterized the organized community explicitly served to enhance their influence.

The primary empirical argument of this work is that the field of nonprofit community-based organizations engaged in HIV/AIDS-related work in New York City developed as a connected community, which I call an urban action network. This network consisted of scores of CBOs, possibly hundreds over the first decade of work, covering a wide range of organizational types, strategies, and relations with state agencies. I view this network as a community of shared meanings and relationships rather than as a formal organizational structure. I therefore used qualitative methods to simultaneously investigate both the forms of exchange among community-based organizations in the HIV/AIDS field and the subjective meaning of those interrelations to the participants. The interorganizational relations were structured, but it is not the structure that particularly interests me.

I propose two claims about this network—first, that the network was constituted out of loose, informal ties, enabling the organized community (or community of organizations) to grow and develop complex interdependencies and informal coordination mechanisms without formal control structures, central points of authority, or a fixed hierarchy. Although the network had no central point of oversight, and hence no one to design its structure, the informal arrangement appears to reflect an intelligence at work. The various groups engaged in a continuous process of negotiation among themselves and between their communities and the state over the nature, meaning, and extent of the HIV/AIDS crisis. The fluidity of the identity of the "AIDS community" allowed the groups to maintain a functional uncertainty in state-community relations. This uncertainty warded off the processes of routinization and institutionalization that so often fix the upper limit on the influence of a community mobilization.

The second claim is that this interorganizational structure is not unique among political mobilizations, but rather that the conditions under which it grew make this case more ideally typical of the form than most. The scope and urgency of the crisis fostered an accelerated, strategically directed, and relatively unimpeded development of community-based work. Additional factors contributed to this growth pattern, including the extent of resources available to organizers in New York; the lethal nature of the crisis, which compelled large numbers of people to mobilize within only a few years; and the prior experience of organizers with activism for women's rights, gay rights, civil rights, and peace. Yet those factors alone are not unique to HIV/AIDS organizing, or even to organizing in New York City, where an unusual density of activists and organizations may be found. Unlike comparable cases, however, this new mobilization experienced a unique amount of "slack." That is to say, the various agencies and interest groups constituting the institutional environment—in this case, state agencies in health and human services, research, and appropriations—failed to form a strong agenda of their own to compete with the community-based HIV/AIDS agenda for nearly ten years. This less-than-benign neglect created unusual organizational conditions in which the work of private organizations was not effectively channeled or co-opted by state institutions in a consistent or overwhelming fashion until the early 1990s.

MEASURING INFORMAL NETWORKING

This book comes at the end of three waves of research. Data are based on multiple phases of fieldwork: research on community-based HIV/AIDS organizations in New York conducted from 1994 to 1997; fieldwork among New York City syringe exchange programs from 1998 to 2000; and comparative research among HIV/AIDS groups in New York and Amsterdam in the summer of 1994 and the fall of 1999.

The findings incorporate information from forty-two community-based organizations in New York City. This number might give the reader a sense that the examination was exhaustive and complete. In fact, one can identify nearly one hundred additional organizations that were not included that reasonably could have been. Nonetheless, there is reason to believe that this large sample represents the field as well as one could. The interviews and other data exhibit coherence and continuity with respect to significant events and moments. Where there are significant disagreements or inconsistencies, these are noted in the text.

Data collection took the form of a multiorganizational ethnography. (See the afterword for more details.) Primary data on community-based organizations comes from both individual and group sources. Fieldwork included interviews with over fifty volunteers and staff; volunteer work for community events; site visits where services were offered; participation in marches, rallies, and funerals;[1] and over one hundred hours of participation in group meetings. Organizational definitions, missions, priorities, and changes were most often documented by the groups themselves in flyers, pamphlets, annual reports, and official websites. Informants addressed attitudes, strategies, internal and external responses to events and plans, and interorganizational dynamics. Secondary sources concerning the study organizations included books and articles written by participants, founders, and directors of the groups as well as media coverage of some of the events or groups discussed.

The organizational histories presented here are therefore often recreations based on conversations after the fact and texts written either during or after the events described. These data are supplemented by admixtures of the two—participant memoirs. Several of the founding organizers in the HIV/ AIDS field have written their own personal histories, and many have contributed papers to conferences and edited books. (The present work was also limited by the fact that at least two informants withheld certain details because they were working on their own books.)

I do not make any attempt to formalize the "true state" of the organizations during the time of the research. I do not record the number of clients served, the identities of funders, or the salaries of executive directors.[2] I seek to measure organizational behavior as it pertains to changes in the groups' missions, priorities, strategies, and interorganizational relations.

Unless otherwise noted, all quotes are taken from interviews conducted by the author with staff or volunteers at HIV/AIDS CBOs. To protect confidentiality, I generally have not used informants' names in this book, either real or pseudonymous. Approximately sixty informants from many locations within the field contributed to the present analysis, each speaking to his own HIV/ AIDS career and experience.[3] Few of them make any claim to officially represent an organization. Each tells only of the developments in which he or she played a part. Most have worked with multiple organizations; some were no longer attached to any CBO at the time of data collection.

The collective identity of a field of organizations as a community is enacted and reproduced through a series of interorganizational relations wherein individuals circulate and wherein knowledge and material resources and other forms of social capital (Coleman 1988; Lin 2001) are exchanged among the community groups. Thus, the unit of analysis is organizational, though the fieldwork and interviews necessarily involve individual social actors who may or may not claim to speak on behalf of a group. In order to measure interorganizational relations using individual histories, informants were asked about moments of network growth, differentiation, realignment, or consolidation. Four types of relations emerged early in the first study and became the focal point of further research: collaboration, referrals, origins, and sponsorship. Each reveals a different aspect of social capital as a resource in motion within a mutually reinforcing social network (Lin 2001; Portes 1998).

The term *collaboration* may be taken to imply formal interorganizational processes such as coalitions and consortia. Given the empirical focus of this work on informal relations, I avoided using this term during the interviews. Instead, informants were asked to identify other organizations that they "worked with" on a fairly routine basis. Informants were also asked to identify other groups or agencies that helped or hindered them in their efforts at any given time. This language encouraged participants to reflect on the kinds of events that brought multiple CBOs together for brief periods out of shared interest. It also led to an indication of which organizations were most visible or interactive in the field, and how others viewed them.

Interorganizational *referrals* likewise have both formal and informal incarnations. The formal variety includes linkage agreements and subcontracting arrangements among service providers. With or without contracts, referrals also function as a form of endorsement. Community-based organizations that send their clients to other agencies are implicitly or explicitly extending the umbrella of their own credibility and reputation to cover the other groups. By the same process, agencies whose interests, accomplishments, or forms are inconsistent with the trends of the field of work are less likely to receive referrals from other groups. Informants in client-service capacities were asked to identify the agencies to which they most frequently referred clients or those to whom they preferred to send clients. They were also asked to identify the agencies or contacts from whom they routinely received clients by referral. Sources at other agencies were asked to identify other agencies that they would personally recommend for various HIV/AIDS needs. The resulting data on referral relations include both the routine organizational practices that many groups adopted, some of which were published in community resource guides, and the personal contacts unique to each informant.

The question of *origins* attempts to measure the organizational context out of which each organization grew, with particular attention to the locations of the founders in the field of work. Some groups began as projects within other organizations. Some emerged as a reaction against the limitations of known groups. Others simply filled newly identified gaps in the field without reference to specific preexisting organizations. Similarly, some organizational founders learned the ropes working with various agencies in a field before putting their own vision into practice, while others who achieved proficiency and experience in unrelated areas of work imported their perspectives and skills into new leadership positions within the field. The latter case also defines the situations of "outside managers" brought in to replace the original founders.

Finally, many organizations explicitly chose to participate in community-building activities by sharing resources, giving grants, or sharing liability and responsibility with other groups on their applications for external support. Such *sponsorship* activities identify the sponsored group as a member of the community (of organizations) that the sponsoring group is seeking to build. Collectively, these four forms of interorganizational relations connect the organizations of this study into a dense web of exchange and, for the most part, support.

Individuals tell their own stories. Weaving the results into a single account is a creative act. The information presented here is as empirically sound and subject to verification as I could manage. I make no claim to have a better or more complete truth than any other version that has been written, and I take responsibility onto myself for any inaccuracies or misrepresentations that may eventually come to light.

PLAN OF THE BOOK

This book, like so many things, is divided into three parts. The first section introduces the theoretical model on which the book is based, the nature of the study, the historical and political context of the events, and the claims that I am making about networks, fields, and contentious politics.

The middle section, the body of the book, tells the story of the groups under discussion, their histories, goals, actions, and interactions. I examine the pattern of emergence of each new area of activity within the field. In telling these stories, I emphasize two aspects from the informants' accounts: the relations between the new organizations and the existing organizations of the field and the shifting configuration of state-community relations. Since my concern is with the unfolding culture and structure of the field of nonprofits, I do not attempt to measure the response of the field's various targets in government or industry. The exception to this is my attempt, in chapter 6, to analyze the process through which the informally constituted field of community-based NPOs gave way to a formally structured, state-centered network.

In the last section, I address the relationship of this case to the general processes of campaigns for social change. It is here that I will argue for a multi-organizational approach to the study of contentious politics.

This introductory chapter defines some terms and distinguishes the organizational, identity-oriented, and public health perspectives on HIV/AIDS. Chapter 1 then establishes the social and political context in which the organizations operated. Most importantly, these chapters seek to define state and community-based action in terms of the relationship between actors in those two sectors. I will argue that it is the nature of this relationship, more than any other single factor, that determined the shape of the responses to HIV/AIDS in New York City and the United States.

Chapter 2 discusses the initial organizational efforts—the elaboration of a new field of action out of the intersection of political, health, and cultural concerns. Beginning with the efforts of the first groups to "do something," this chapter follows the early explorations of what community groups should do, and it ends with the formation of new CBOs dedicated to the creation of an empowerment movement for people with HIV/AIDS. In this phase of community organizing, from 1981 to about 1986, the community gradually moved from an uncertain quest for information to an organized campaign for recognition. They made HIV/AIDS an event around which to mobilize and proffered their own definitions of the affected peoples.

Chapters 3 and 4 examine organizing efforts by, for, or directed at communities of color and other relatively disenfranchised groups from the mid-1980s until the early 1990s. The tension of this wave of activity recapitulates much of the tension inherent in all identity politics. Non-White groups were defined as "different," and this difference can be both marginalizing and empowering. Organizational efforts on behalf of people of color that were too derivative of, or generated by, efforts that began in either predominantly White communities or government agencies were not culturally specific, appropriate, or sensitive to the situations and interests of the target populations. At the same time, communities of color were able to form alliances with mostly White community-based organizations that had preceded them in the HIV/AIDS field. Chapter 3 addresses these processes for most of the affected communities that mobilized in the middle of the decade. Chapter 4 examines the same story for community groups concerned with HIV/AIDS among drug users, which also began work far outside of the organized community before integrating into the existing field. These alliances—of community groups, independent of the state—strengthened the community overall and increased the influence and legitimacy of community-based claims making against government agencies. This period of activity greatly broadened both public and local discourse on the nature and meaning of HIV/AIDS. In so doing, it extended the working definition of who was represented or not within the "AIDS community."

Chapter 5 returns to the mid- to late 1980s in order to trace the development of one of the most unique and influential paths of community organizing in the response to HIV/AIDS: from the organizational efforts of the empowerment movement, through the patient-as-expert campaigns, to political activism, to treatment activism. Treatment activism was not the endpoint of political activism around HIV/AIDS by any means. But, I argue, it had the greatest impact on the nature of relations between the state and the community. Treatment activism is offered as evidence of the complete restructuring of relations between the two sectors accomplished by the efforts of the activists and as a new dimension of the state-community partnership around HIV/AIDS that was more than a few years in the making.

Finally, chapter 6 ends the social history of the HIV/AIDS field with a metaevaluation of the multiagency service consortia supported by the Ryan White Comprehensive AIDS Resources Emergency Act of 1990. This formal interorganizational system of relations simultaneously brought the experience of the community and the resources of the state into cities that lacked coordinated responses to HIV/AIDS. Almost overnight, it replaced the informal urban action network that had grown in New York with a state-centered model. I will use this model to elaborate on the factors that made the community model unique. This chapter ends with a brief summary of changes in the world of HIV/AIDS in the decade since the institutionalizing of AIDS work.

In the last section, I return to questions of organizing collective action. Chapter 7 formalizes and generalizes the urban action network model. The conclusion offers speculations based upon this study for the understanding of contentious politics and organizational fields in the era of globalization. This chapter also contains some speculative conclusions concerning community-based organizing and the bartering of influence in state-centered policy processes. I end there with a brief return to the concept of an organized community.

NOTES

1. In HIV/AIDS activism, funerals may be protest events, and many were scheduled "political funerals."

2. Attempts by others to collect more rigorous data on organizational details and linkages in the nonprofit sector using surveys and self-reports have suffered from low response rates. See Blau and Rabenovic (1991).

3. The imprecision in the number of sources reflects the variety of forms of participation. Forty-five formal interviews were supplemented by dozens of short, informative conversations and clarifications as well as e-mail exchanges, some during the period of writing, long after the fieldwork had been completed.

Part One

RESPONDING TO HIV/AIDS

Chapter One

Formal and Informal Responses, 1981–1991

For those who were aware of HIV/AIDS in the United States during the early 1980s, the cognitive dissonance was reminiscent of *The Invasion of the Body Snatchers*. All around them, friends and loved ones were being struck down without warning or apparent cause. But officially, as far as their doctors or newspapers were reporting, nothing was happening. There were no visible public health mobilizations, no widespread warnings, and no apparent concern.

In fact, a great deal was happening, but quietly, in the margins of social life and on the margins of epidemiological research. A response was building, linking individuals, groups, patients, doctors, and families in a recognizable new field of work. An uncoordinated but growing community mobilization was forging a web of connections surrounding, but rarely penetrating, the institutional centers of the public heath sector. A network of outsiders was creating an organized public space, a resistance movement almost, from which to challenge AIDS in their midst.

Within government and public health institutions, the response to HIV/ AIDS was shaped by the ascribed identity characteristics of those most affected, characteristics that necessarily diminished the status of the condition and its sufferers. The early epidemiology of HIV/AIDS was dominated by "lifestyle" hypotheses, which, despite the incidents of heterosexual AIDS and inconsistent patterns of drug use among gay patients, focused excessively on gay sexuality and popular club drugs (Oppenheimer 1988). Doctors who attempted to treat and learn from AIDS patients sometimes faced pressure to stop doing so for fear that their hospitals would gain a welcoming reputation among sick, gay men. HIV/AIDS work was described as a special interest, not a "legitimate area of medical inquiry" (Shilts 1987, 169). This distinction may not have been entirely careless. "AIDS is not only stigmatized, but expensive," as Anthony Lemelle and Charlene Harrington point out. "The reproduction of stigma associated with AIDS is of paramount importance for the reproduction of privilege in terms of class, gender, and race. By relegating the victims of AIDS to the category of 'Other' with moral deficiencies, it makes the idea of overlooking their medical caregiving needs more palatable to a nation ostensibly committed to promoting the general welfare" (1998, 162).

The language used to discuss HIV/AIDS outside of community settings was one of the most striking aspects of the marginalizing process. In 1983, the Centers for Disease Control and Prevention (CDC) identified population categories in which HIV/AIDS cases seemed, without explanation, to be clustering and labeled them as "risk groups" (CDC 1983b). In conversation and public documents, the term was used in contrast to the "general population" (Oppenheimer 1988, 60). "Soon, members of these groups were popularly termed 'the Four-H Club,' a shorthand reference to homosexuals, Haitians, hemophiliacs and heroin-users" (Farmer 1992, 211). The initial CDC report contained a few qualifications but did not give any clear guidelines for estimating what percentage of a population constituted a risk group. With its gratuitous use of terms like "illicit" and "abusers," the article implied moral culpability without explicitly discussing causality. The news media could hardly be blamed for treating the risk-group designation as AIDS "vectors," contaminated groups whose presence threatened "the rest of us." Based on the CDC designation, the Public Health Service issued its first HIV/AIDS prevention guidelines: Gay men should have fewer sexual partners and that no one in a risk group should donate blood (Curran 1986).

The specific advice had merit, but it showed far less concern with how those at risk could protect themselves than with how those most likely to be contaminated could avoid affecting everybody else. The designations of risk groups rather than risk behaviors encouraged the popular misconception that HIV/AIDS was a problem of deviant people, a disease that had naturally selected and thereby revealed the unclean among us. Twenty-five years later, it is difficult to recall that moral and political leaders claimed that HIV/AIDS was a punishment from God against sinners (Hallett and Cannella 1994), and that proposals for quarantine camps were actually discussed in the mainstream news media (Kinsella 1989). As Robert Padgug then wrote, "various forms of expulsion—real and symbolic—from society as a whole and, especially, from the realm of politics and public discourse have been proposed: quarantine and other forms of isolation for AIDS sufferers, public surveillance of HIV-positive individuals, HIV antibody testing without sufficient provision for confidentiality or anonymity, the general refusal to discuss homosexual sex acts publicly, as well as the strong desire of much of the population to remove AIDS patients from schools, jobs, and housing" (1987, 296).

The main problem with the language of "risk groups," as Rose Weitz (1991) discussed, was that it confused behavior with identity. "Gay men" were a risk group, and so gay men were perceived, labeled, and treated as carriers either of disease or of an undefined propensity to disease. This obscuring of the mode of transmission—unprotected intercourse—created and propagated a number of myths and misunderstandings that were deeply antithetical to public health interests. First, by focusing on the identity characteristic rather than on the behavior, the label encouraged hostility, fear, and discrimination against gay men and other "risk groups." Had the discourse been on behavior, it could have alleviated the fears of neighbors and coworkers whose contact with individual homosexual men was casual at best. More importantly, the misidentification of risk groups helped to foster a mistaken sense of safety among heterosexuals who were encouraged to think of HIV/AIDS as a disease that affected "other people" (Treichler 1988). Further, as Simon Watney (1987) argued, the distinction between risk groups and the so-called general public often served as a thin cover for a hostile moral contrast of homosexuality itself versus "the family." The language of groups, which moralizes the distinction between those who are inherently at risk from those who aren't, introduced powerful new reasons not to engage in safer sex. To ask for or offer a condom suggests that one of the partners is in the "other" group. In extreme cases, women have been beaten by their sexual partners for wanting to use a condom on the pretext that the suggestion was a moral slight against the man (Anastos and Marte 1991).

The concept of a risk group and its accompanying culture of risky behaviors also limited epidemiological research and research on interventions. Even in cases where social scientists have attempted to focus HIV/AIDS discourse on political, social, or economic structures, health researchers and others have often redirected the conversation back to "the cultures of high-risk groups" (Glick Schiller 2002, 238).

And finally, the almost willful refusal to discuss sexual behaviors, particularly "deviant" ones, undermined the early attempts to do HIV prevention education. Numerous studies have affirmed that both heterosexuals and homosexuals willingly altered their sexual behaviors once they understood what the virus was and how it was transmitted (Aggleton 1997; Freudenberg 1990; Kelly and St. Lawrence 1990). Unfortunately, misinformation and denial were as common as prevention education, including a famous 1988 *Cosmopolitan* article telling the target readership of presumably straight White women not to let the HIV/AIDS hype spoil their sex lives, since it didn't really threaten them (Joseph 1992, 142). Similar contradictions have been identified concerning prevention efforts directed toward injecting drug users (IDUs). Despite evidence that IDUs were also willing and able to reduce risk once the means were made available (Heckathorn et al. 1999; van den Hoek et al. 1989), coercive interventions were preferred over harm reduction ones, due in part to the negative imagery associated with drug users (Des Jarlais et al. 2000, 161). Within clinical literature, the population was often described as "disaffiliated" and chaotic abusers with no social sensibility (Crystal and Glick Schiller 1993), while the popular press favored sensational stories of drug-related violence and the crack "epidemic" (Reinarman and Levine 1997).

Looking back, we can distinguish between the health issues and the political and social issues circumscribing the lives of those affected by HIV/AIDS. The health issues were primarily behavioral, for HIV is a virus transmitted through specific acts involving the exchange of blood or semen. Potential transmission vectors are created during sexual encounters, fights, childbirth, blood transfusions, injections, and many other circumstances, without regard for the identities or culpability of the people involved. Politically and socially, however, the discourse on HIV/AIDS was all about exclusionary identities. Prevention education that acknowledged that men had sex with men was denounced in Congress as "gay pornography." Syringe exchange programs, which have been the only interventions to significantly reduce the spread of HIV among drug injectors worldwide, remain illegal in much of the United States even now on the grounds that they "send the wrong message" to drug users and America's youth (ONDCP 1999; Whitman 1998). The first attempts to establish exchange sites in New York in 1988 were denounced as "genocidal" policies designed to increase drug use among the African American population (W. Anderson 1991, 1506). The public and political fetishization of the identities of those most at risk diverted our attention from the dissemination of useful information and practical interventions toward the distinction between the "innocent victims" and the guilty. The language we used, and even the data we collected, reinforced the marginal social status of HIV/AIDS.

Although HIV/AIDS had been found among drug injectors as early as 1981, the popular conception of the syndrome, among those few who knew of it at all, was that of a "gay cancer." Even after epidemiologists had modeled the condition as a blood-borne agent, most likely a sexually transmitted virus, with other paths unknown (Curran 1986, xxii), researchers and science writers still referred to AIDS as "Gay-Related Immune Deficiency," or GRID, with very little specification of how, exactly, the etiology was related to homosexuality. (One early AIDS researcher contrasted the "vulnerable rectum" to the "rugged vagina," but for the most part it was enough to know that homosexuality itself was part of the problem.) When injecting drug users began to receive attention, they were inevitably referred to in the media and in government documents as "drug abusers," as they still are. Yet drug abuse, per se, is not the risk factor. It is the needle, not the drug—the commingled blood, not the illegality of the act—that placed them at risk for HIV transmission.

STATE-CENTERED RESPONSES TO HIV/AIDS

Within governmental circles, those most responsible for forming a national AIDS strategy demonstrated a consistent inability to commit to one. Presidents Ronald Reagan and George H. W. Bush, who between them occupied the White House throughout the first twelve years of the epidemic, each convened advisory commissions to recommend federal policies. Neither implemented the majority of the recommendations. The first panel was established in 1987 under the leadership of Eugene Mayberry, who resigned the following year citing lack of administrative support (Malinowsky and Perry 1991, 3). The commission's report, issued in 1988, criticized the Reagan administration for lack of leadership and called for sweeping changes in HIV/AIDS care, outreach to drug users, increased investment in drug treatment, and new health care initiatives for the poor and uninsured (Presidential Commission on the HIV Epidemic 1988). The same report faulted the public health sector for failing to work with community-based physicians, gave credit to community-based organizations (CBOs) for leading the nation's response to the epidemic, and urged the administration to support the work of the organized communities. None of these recommendations was adopted. Later that year, the National Academy of Sciences issued its own report on federal HIV/AIDS policies, also criticizing the administration for its lack of leadership. The following year, the scenario was repeated as President Bush's advisory commission issued its report calling the federal response to HIV/AIDS inadequate and repeating many of the same recommendations of the previous commission. A few years later, a further presidential commission found state and federal responses "glacially slow," leaving community-based organizations to cover the most "desperately needed services" (Presidential Commission on HIV 1992, 116). Following each of the reports, the administrations that had commissioned them consistently rejected or ignored the majority of the reports' recommendations.

School boards throughout the country received widespread media attention and general public support for barring children with AIDS from attending classes, or for requiring them to use separate bathrooms, stay away from water fountains, and carry their own disposable utensils, as was the case for Ryan White in Indiana (Kirp 1989, 51). In one notorious Florida case, after three HIV-positive children had already been forced out of school by the local community, their house was burned down by arsonists (Doka 1997, 69). As the public's awareness of AIDS increased, particularly following the death of Rock Hudson in 1985, incidents of job and housing discrimination rose dramatically. Gallup polls during the period from 1987 to 1988 revealed popular approval for these acts, despite their illegality (Blendon and Donelan 1990). As late as 1993, the National Commission on AIDS characterized the national response as "a decade of unreasoning fear and cruel indifference" (National Commission on AIDS 1993, 1). Beginning in San Francisco in 1985, numerous local districts and eventually most states responded by enacting anti–AIDS discrimination legislation. While the first presidential commission and other panels repeatedly recommended such measures, then-president Reagan opposed federal discrimination legislation. In 1988, the president vetoed the Civil Rights Restoration Act, which had contained protections against AIDS discrimination. The veto was overridden by Congress.

A further governmental pattern throughout the first decade concerned HIV/AIDS funding. Once AIDS had been identified as a budgetary item of its own, the Reagan and Bush administrations' budget proposals consistently and significantly undercut the amounts requested by the National Institutes of Health and the Public Health Service, placing Congress in the unusual position of allocating far greater sums than had been requested by the White House (Perrow and Guillèn 1990). On several occasions, the Reagan administration sought to cut AIDS spending that had already been approved. Even the 1990 Ryan White Comprehensive AIDS Emergency Resources (CARE) Act, which presently funds the majority of coordinated HIV/AIDS services in the United States, passed over the objections of President Bush. The National Commission on AIDS Working Group on Social and Human Issues noted in its 1991 report that "although the legislation was overwhelmingly supported by Congress, it has been appropriated at a level far short of what had originally been anticipated, far short of what is needed" (Working Group on Social and Human Issues 1991). At that point, the CARE Act funding had yet to be released. Approved as an emergency measure in 1990, disbursement of support for the CARE Act's "disaster relief" measures was further delayed until 1992 (Chambré 1996, 162).

If the relative lack of formal actions against HIV/AIDS raised suspicions among activists that the government did not consider the epidemic to be a priority, numerous legislative measures appeared to specifically threaten people affected by AIDS. In 1983, the community organization that would later become AIDS Project Los Angeles (APLA) completed the nation's first prevention materials on safer sex, which included instructions for condom use during anal sex and alternatives to penetrative sex. The Los Angeles County Supervisors, who had sponsored the materials, refused to allow their distribution, calling the recommendations pornography that "attempts to subsidize deviant behavior" (Malinowski and Perry 1991, 4). Subsequently, the State of California "created a Materials Review Committee which recommended that 'it is preferable to use clinical or descriptive terms describing sexual contact or behavior . . . rather than their slang or "street language equivalents"'" (Bayer and Kirp 1992, 35), thereby officially rejecting community-based AIDS prevention materials that actively targeted communities at risk on their own terms. Federal policy makers then went one step further in directing that "any health information developed by the federal government . . . should encourage responsible sexual behavior . . . based on fidelity, commitment, maturity, [and] placing sexuality within the context of marriage" (Bayer and Kirp 1992, 35, quoting Edwin Meese III, memorandum for the Domestic Policy Council [February 11, 1987]). This restriction effectively stipulated that AIDS prevention education material should not acknowledge or address the existence of homosexuality or multiple sexual partners. Speaking at the International Conference on AIDS that year, John D'Eramo of Gay Men's Health Crisis (GMHC) declared that "the prohibition of frank language in AIDS prevention is ridiculous, and AIDS organizations who accept government funding which requires this 'polite' talk have truly sold their collective souls" (D'Eramo 1987, 259). Nonetheless, organizations such as GMHC did rely on government funds and generally adhered to the provisions.

Finally, and most dramatically, the Helms Amendment in 1987 forbade federal funding for any HIV/AIDS-related initiative, including prevention education or targeted outreach materials that could be construed as condoning or "promoting" homosexuality. "Enraged by a sexually explicit 'safer-sex' comic book produced by the New York City–based Gay Men's Health Crisis, a recipient of federal funds, [Jesse] Helms denounced the 'promotion of sodomy' by the government" (Bayer and Kirp 1992, 36). Known to activists as the "No Promo Homo" Act, the Helms Amendment implied that the threat of HIV/ AIDS was of less concern than the danger that gays would feel accepted in American society. Despite indications that this position was a minority one in Congress, the measure passed with overwhelming approval and little dissent.

As we look back, the inadequacy of the government response seems now to have been a systemic failure exacerbated by uncertainty, inconsistency, and a general lack of urgency rather than any agreed-upon policy of neglect. Many political leaders took individual action against HIV/AIDS, and community advocates found supporters at all but the highest levels of government. And while no significant legislation specifically designed to help people with HIV/AIDS was introduced by Congress until the tenth year of the epidemic, they were able to prevent massive cuts in funding and the gutting of helpful programs that had started elsewhere. Collectively, however, the public health sector was not prepared to deal with HIV/AIDS without a significant reorganization and an unambiguous mandate, neither of which was forthcoming under an administration that had promised vast reductions in federal spending and that received much of its support from the religious right (Perrow and Guillén 1990).

At the state and local level, HIV/AIDS issues received a slightly better hearing. A 1989 survey of state health officials and legislators found that most of the respondents considered their states' responses to be fair but not impressive (Backstrom and Robins 1995). The authors of that study reported that while policy makers relied more on the recommendations of health officials than on other sources for policy guidance, none aggressively pursued the complete agendas proposed by their health departments. Many elected officials defined their greatest legislative accomplishments as the prevention of particularly harmful or punishing proposals targeted against people with HIV/AIDS rather than the enactment of anything more proactive. The same study found that state governors tended to avoid personal involvement in HIV/AIDS issues and were happy to allow their health departments to take full responsibility for policy in this arena. In sum, the formal responses to HIV/AIDS during the first ten years of the epidemic were unimpressive, insufficient, and inconsistent.

COMMUNITY-BASED RESPONSES TO HIV/AIDS

Community-based responses to HIV/AIDS, whether organized or not, either took their lead from or reacted against the tone set by the federal government. Activists and advocates for people living with HIV/AIDS have often portrayed government agencies as their enemies. The government's failure to stop HIV/AIDS early on, or even to develop a plan, particularly exacerbated longstanding conflicts between the state and people of color. Proponents of "planned shrinkage" arguments suggested that the state did not mind the idea of a plague that targeted gays, the poor, and minorities, and that we would see a more concerted response when it reached the "general population" (Wallace 1992). Invoking the legacy of the Tuskegee syphilis experiments that, with the complicity of the Public Health Service and the army, caused several hundred African American men and their partners to face illness or death, leaders questioned the integrity of the few public health interventions that targeted minority communities (Thomas and Quinn 1991). African American politicians, organizers, and writers denounced proposals such as free condom distribution and syringe exchange programs as "genocidal" schemes to further reduce minority populations or to encourage drug "slavery" (Quimby 1993, 219).

The powerful association between a frightening new medical condition and sexual identity labels engendered two related responses that would establish the course of responses to HIV/AIDS outside of the San Francisco Bay Area for the next ten years. Researchers, particularly those in the government research institutions and leading universities, avoided HIV/AIDS work, partially out of fear of being tainted with the stigma of homosexuality (Galatowitch 1996). HIV/AIDS work raised questions about researchers' priorities, which generated a fear of being outed or of being assumed gay. This was equally true, or even more threatening, for openly lesbian and gay scientists who were continuously negotiating their sexual identities and their professional identities with the vagaries of these institutional prejudices (Galatowitch 1996; Perrow and Guillèn 1990). (Public health officials in San Francisco, after years of close involvement with a politically involved gay community, did not have to fear this "courtesy stigma" to the same extent [Silverman 1987].) On the other hand, within gay urban enclaves, informal community leaders were called to action by the notion of a deadly disease that "targeted" gay men. And if they were mobilized at all by the presence of HIV/AIDS in their communities, they were incensed and outraged by the apparent lack of concern from all other quarters. The first one hundred deaths were terrifying enough to those who noted them, but even after the first one thousand, no centrally coordinated response had emerged from the public health sector. The silence itself formed the target of early writings on HIV/AIDS. The death toll rose most quickly in New York City, where Larry Kramer's 1983 article "1,112 and Counting" went largely unnoticed beyond the readership of *The New York Native*, a gay newspaper. In cities with fewer cases and no gay media, even Kramer's writings were relatively unknown.

Community-Based Organizing

The HIV/AIDS action network in New York City grew as a greater variety of independently constituted communities came to accept AIDS as a threat to their own members. Despite governmental and media framing of HIV/AIDS first as a gay disease and later as a problem of special interest groups—not affecting "the general population"—many communities came together in shared ownership of the issue. The early risers in the gay community accomplished a great deal in education and outreach, but on their own they had only limited success in gaining access to political processes. The organized community's efforts on multiple fronts, operating through multiple venues that involved a variety of private and governmental agencies, created a complex set of alliances and antagonisms between the state and the community. By dynamically manipulating these relations, the organized community penetrated deep into the state's HIV/AIDS policy arena.

Organizing around something often entails organizing against someone (Lune 2002b). Diverse groups can find unity in their opposition to someone else even in the absence of stronger ties among themselves. In a political context, popular mobilizations rely on "the construction of group boundaries that establish differences between a challenging group and dominant groups" (Taylor and Whittier 1995, 173). In the case of HIV/AIDS, legislators and policy makers made this process easier, having defined themselves as dominant and the communities of affected people as marginal, without actually establishing a dominant course of action.

The AIDS-related community-based organizations (CBOs) implicitly or explicitly built a wall of resistance against the "outside" forces that sought to imprint their own stigmatizing identity constructs onto the affected peoples (Siegel, Lune, and Meyers 1998). Broadly conceived labels for socially constructed identities such as "people living with HIV/AIDS" are more abstract and elusive than seemingly essentialist identity aspects such as gender and ethnicity. Correspondingly, the field of HIV/AIDS organizations contained lines of fragmentation based on demographic categories. Such divisions also provided points of contention in debates over such issues as the "fair share of the pie" in public funding, which pitted the so-called poor-Black groups against the downtown-gay-White-male CBOs (*Poz Magazine* 1997). Nonetheless, the differences between groups within the field are less salient and less precise than the differences between the field of community-based organizations and the institutions of the state or industry. Participants in the CBOs distinguished their work and their interests from that of the state-centered institutions of the sectors in which their work is embedded and from the interests and efforts of the pharmaceutical industry (Lune and Oberstein 2001).

Within any diverse organizational field, one will encounter struggles over resources and power (Galatowitch 1996; Klandermans 1992; Perrow and Guillén 1990). One may view these struggles as impediments to developing a coherent community-based strategy (Patton 1990). Nonetheless, given the complex nature of the identity conflicts engendered by HIV/AIDS, both within and beyond the active gay communities, such conflicts are inevitable. Yet such conditions make the question of organized cooperation even more essential. How can the individual members of a diverse organizational field function integratively? What holds the field together?

URBAN ACTION NETWORKS

I define an urban action network as a nonprofit, interorganizational structure located within a bounded geographical space and defined around an area of collective action or a "policy domain" (Burstein 1991). The term "action network" indicates a shared structure and hence a related background or some shared history coupled with the intent to do something. The action component emphasizes the inclusion of activists and advocates within the network. Among the various forms of action pertinent to a policy domain will be attempts to forcibly alter or shape policy. Yet we cannot judge the entire network in terms of social movement activism. Other forms of action can include education and community outreach, legal and medical advocacy, service provision, consciousness raising, research, and fundraising. Each of these forms of work has an influence on the three major aspects of the policy process: "agenda setting, the development of policy proposals, and the struggle for adoption of particular proposals" (Burstein 1991, 327). An urban action network, therefore, likely contains but is not coterminous with an urban social movement.

Sharing a history or other cultural connections in no way implies that members of the network will share a single vision of the best approach to the forms and tactics of the collective action—far from it. The network structure implies diverse elements that are bound by fluid connections but yet are not subservient to a hierarchy. Such a relational system provides the terrain in which diverse organizations can interact without surrendering their independence, their diversity, or their disagreements. At the same time, as a single organizational unit, the network provides a shared space in which collective identities can be negotiated. The dynamic processes cannot be reasonably explained only in terms of the goals or practices of individual organizations, however dominant one group might be at any moment. The linkages that the groups form, and the further relations that develop through these linkages, serve the network as a network or the community as a community, even at the expense of organizations that initiate these relations.

Structurally, the interorganizational relations of an urban action network resemble the forms described by Luther Gerlach and Virginia Hine (1970) as segmentary, polycephalous networks. As with this form, urban action networks are interorganizational networks of relatively independent clusters (segments), with no single point of control (multiheaded), with routine interactions. The Gerlach and Hine model, however, referred to relations among organizations within a particular social movement. As such, the interorganizational relations captured by those studies pertained to distinctions and working relations among self-identified social movement organizations involved in a single struggle. By inference, one ought to expect to find a comparable system of relations linking movement organizations with advocacy groups, service providers, educators, and other nonmovement organizations within a policy domain of common interest. To date, however, that proposition has not been empirically tested.

To study a field of organizations and the relations between a field of organizing and a policy sector, I draw upon Russel Curtis and Louis Zurcher's (1975) pioneering work on multiorganizational fields as well as subsequent developments of the notion in social movement studies (Klandermans 1992; Snow, Zurcher, and Ekland-Olson 1980) and neoinstitutional analyses of organizations (DiMaggio and Powell 1983; Jepperson 1991). I have chosen to introduce a slightly different terminology, however, to reflect differences in the perspectives and assumptions of the current study in contrast to these earlier works. Prior studies of interorganizational relations in fields of collective action have addressed questions particular to the growth of social movements with attention to the alignment of consensus around movement frames (Klandermans 1992) and the recruitment of new supporters (Curtis and Zurcher 1975; Snow, Zurcher, and Ekland-Olson 1980). As such, these authors examined networking from the perspective of a focal movement organization with the rest of the field comprising "both supportive and antagonistic" (Klandermans 1992) organizations and interest groups that could be found to contribute to, or to detract from, the framing efforts of the principal social actors. The interorganizational network necessarily contained more groups than the focal social movement organization, but we did not know very much about those other groups. This line of research invites us to generalize the processes beyond the assumptions pertinent to social movement studies and beyond the effects on a focal organization. The present work, therefore, examines the growth and development of a particular kind of organizational field in which contentious politics may occur but need not, in which the field itself rather than any focal group is the unit of analysis. Although this study draws upon research on collective action and contentious politics, I seek to shift the focus to the processes of collective organization.

I use the term "urban action network" to define the relational processes characterizing the workings of the organized HIV/AIDS community. We may apply the term as an ideal type of an informally constituted interorganizational network capable of growth, coordination, and political action without a centralized control structure. This composition of interorganizational relations allows and encourages multivocality and the simultaneous pursuit of multiple campaigns of mutual interest to the participants. The interorganizational network ties together groups within an identifiable field of diverse organizations. It is inherent in the notion of a field that the network comprises nonmovement organizations in addition to any social movement organizations and that the nonmovement groups are not considered only as the support system for the movement activity. Urban action networks engage multiple organizations and constituencies in a variety of semicoordinated actions within a single policy domain.

The organizational field may be conceived of as a space of work. In Paul DiMaggio and Walter Powell's classic formulation, an "organizational field" refers to "those organizations that, in the aggregate, constitute a recognized area of institutional life" (1983, xx). Although an organizational field is structured by interorganizational linkages, DiMaggio and Powell's use of the term is more cultural than structural. The field exists as a field because the shared area of work is recognized as such, not because the groups in the field achieve any particular density of connectedness or frequency of exchange. Interorganizational networking occurs within an organizational field, but the field is not inherently defined by it. People, information, and other resources flow throughout the field, overlaying a variety of network structures on the otherwise open space. Social actors—organizations—within the network have channels of access to each other, whether they use them or not. Organized action by network actors affects not only the acting group and its members, but the rest of the organized community as well. An organization that strikes a new deal with state regulators or that engages in a new level of civil disobedience alters the nature of the relations between the entire network of community-based organizations and its environment, whether they do so as part of a long-term strategy or as an isolated act. To the extent that the network consolidates—as the density of connections increases—there will be more opportunities for strategizing at the collective level or with a greater awareness of the impact of actions throughout the field.

An urban action network is not confined to a single form of action. Within its contours, activists, advocates, service providers, writers, researchers, patients, and therapists (or tenants and lawyers, as the case may be) interact, coordinate, and collide. What they share is a domain of work such as HIV/AIDS, a community constituency, which includes physical proximity as well as shared issues or grievances, and a set of targets such as the state or an industry. There are events of interest to the community and events created by the community. Through planning, advertising, or participating in these events, members of the organized community cross paths. By sharing information and other resources and by collaborating, strategizing, or negotiating, organizational leaders also come together around issues of mutual concern. Implicitly, an interorganizational network will come to be suffused with interpersonal networks.

Within the shared space of an organizational field, there is no need to share a single goal or strategy. As a networked space, however, the field provides the organizational framework for ongoing discussions and explorations of shared goals, multiple strategies, and a distributed awareness of multiple interests. Whereas an organization in the network will be formally dedicated to the pursuit of a specific goal, organizational participants will need to have an awareness of the more-or-less related interests of other groups and other population clusters. As one group in the New York City HIV/AIDS network lobbies for more research money for the best and newest treatments for HIV, another organization might press for the wider availability of whatever exists now on behalf of the poorest patient groups who lack access to the highest standards of care. For the two organizations to place their interests in opposition to one another would be a failure of networking. To show awareness of the resources of the network, they might collaborate on certain events. In either case, whether they are self-conscious about their similar locations within the shared space of work or not, the similarity itself predicts that they will be brought into routine contact (Borgatti and Everett 1992).

In chapter 2, I trace the origins of the first HIV/AIDS CBOs, the "early risers" (Tarrow 1994) of the community-based mobilization. This chapter will also introduce the earliest interorganizational relations through which the contours of the emerging field of HIV/AIDS organizing were defined. Beginning with a nameless void in 1981, the year of the first identified cases, new community-based organizations had, by 1984, created both an organizational context in which HIV/AIDS services and education could be provided and a conceptual terrain in which future endeavors would take root.

Part Two

COMMUNITY ORGANIZING IN NEW YORK CITY

Chapter Two

A New Field of Work

There were about thirty of us in a comfortable conference room at four in the afternoon. It could have been any business presentation at any corporation. The presenter spoke about the varieties of needs that an HIV-positive person faces, from emotional support to quality medical care. The best treatments available were hard to come by and depended as much on the determination of the patient as on the expertise of the doctor. Some drugs were only available in clinical trials, and their interactions with other drugs were not known. Some could only be taken on a full stomach, others on an empty one. Compliance with complex written instructions was essential, and some doctors would not volunteer all options to their patients unless one had demonstrated the ability to stick with the regimen. People took notes or asked questions, as one would at any professional presentation. But periodically throughout the afternoon, people's watch alarms would beep, and the pillboxes would come out. These were knowledgeable patients, not clinicians. The audience embodied the subject.

Perceptions of HIV/AIDS in the early 1980s were shaped predominantly by reports from the Centers for Disease Control and Prevention (CDC). Community organizing at first followed CDC criteria, generating new organizational efforts for each new crisis area only after it was officially identified. Later, as the community groups gained experience and expertise, they began to define the contours of the problem themselves and to export their definitions and priorities to the public health sector. At the CDC and the National Institutes of Health (NIH), lacking a clear federal mandate or material support, researchers were glad to have the help. "The leadership vacuum from 1981–1985 created the need for another group to define AIDS as a social problem and provide the public with information. . . . While the gay community had to struggle against the stigma of homosexuality (and charismatic right wing leaders) they had little competition in defining the problem by political and medical leaders in the early years" (Cuthbert 1990, 102–3).

Once the field of legitimate expertise began to shift, however, from the scientific world to the organized AIDS community, a new, more self-referential standard emerged in which the logic of experience guided the shape of the work, even to the point of identifying not-yet-at-risk groups for whom advocacy was necessary (Altman 1988; Epstein 1996). The first period of community organizing saw five community-based organizations (CBOs) arise in response to HIV/AIDS in New York City. Each one set out to address HIV/AIDS on behalf of its particular perception of the affected communities. Each drew upon different sources of initial resources, reshaping them to the situation of people living with HIV/AIDS. Each CBO also acted, at first, as though it were at the center of HIV/AIDS work in the city. Interorganizational networking would follow later. Finally, as the participants began to move toward a shared understanding of their communal identity, organized efforts coalesced on claims for group recognition.

HIV/AIDS EARLY RISERS, 1981–1984

GMHC

Three of the new organizations either began as, or quickly reorganized into, service organizations. Gay Men's Health Crisis (GMHC), the first and always the largest, defined itself as *the* AIDS organization. All community services, fundraising, awareness, education, and advocacy occurred under their auspices. They defined AIDS as a gay disease against which gay men must organize for themselves. They organized large fundraisers for medical research and immediately began writing and distributing warning literature for the gay community about a possible new sexually transmitted disease. As their first public service projects, GMHC opened a twenty-four-hour hotline and devised the buddy program, a system of volunteer-based care and service provision by and for members of the self-identified gay community. "At the time, GMHC's hotline was the only source of up-to-date information about AIDS—not that there was much to know; the whole volunteer training manual at the time could have been recorded on a three-by-five card" (Reinfeld 1994, 180).

As the field diversified, GMHC diversified, starting a new program of its own to match virtually every new community initiative. To this day, "work doesn't happen without their presence" (Kayal 1993, 2). An informant referred to the first phone call that so many New Yorkers make upon learning that they are HIV-positive, their call to the GMHC hotline, as "checking in with headquarters." Nonetheless, as their name implied, Gay Men's Health Crisis was firmly entrenched in the gay community. In defining their AIDS-specific role, they drew upon the resources (financial and communicative) of the politically active gay rights movement.

The group's founders were sufficiently rooted in gay politics to start a new community-based organization but without being irrevocably attached to the prior work's ongoing mission and interests. A great deal of the early work by which GMHC organizers defined the domain of AIDS work was antithetical to the "sex positive" messages of the gay rights movement and in fact was often antiliberatory. Community organizers had to define HIV/AIDS as a new problem, distinct from gay politics, that still belonged to the gay community to solve. Their organizational name indicated both the embeddedness of the group in the gay community and their break from identity-oriented sexual politics.

ARC

The AIDS Resource Center (ARC) began operations in the Greenwich Village area in 1983 with a focus on counseling and temporary shelter. ARC brought together "business owners, gay activists, and clergy to provide housing plus practical, emotional and spiritual support to the growing number of homeless people with AIDS (PWAs) living on the streets of New York City" (ARC n.d.). The group's principal founder, Reverend Lee Hancock, worked from the Judson Memorial Baptist Church, but ARC was a neighborhood project.[1] ARC's community was defined geographically but mostly included low-income or homeless people of color, including many drug users. Although ARC's founding was partially gay based, their mission was to care for the homeless and sick who lacked other options. Additionally, as a church-based organization concerned with discrimination against PWAs, ARC created an informal network of pastoral referrals—a hotline of "sympathetic" ministers. ARC invoked a hospice tradition but with a case management model.

ARC sought scatter-site housing for homeless PWAs and established a contract with the city's Human Resources Administration to cover the costs. They demonstrated that a previously undefined need existed, and they established their ability to address it. Having achieved organizational stability and legitimacy within the community and among service providers, they quickly began to develop plans for city-funded service expansions and to seek grants and other support.

HCA

The Haitian Coalition on AIDS (HCA) formed in 1983 as an offshoot of the Haitian Centers Council (HCC, founded in 1982) in Brooklyn, which already had a defined constituency and a working model of community-based social support. They provided Creole and French education material; service coordination; and later, legal advocacy to Haitian residents affected by HIV/AIDS, although a staff member described the organization as having "no boundaries . . . no one agenda." A considerable portion of their attention went toward case management, connecting clients with city entitlements and protecting them from housing, job, and service discrimination. HCA defined as its domain all HIV/AIDS work needed by the Haitian community in New York.

HCA was only partially a response to the relatively high incidence rates among Haitians in New York. The direct trigger was the listing by the CDC of Haitians as an AIDS risk group and the subsequent wave of anti-Caribbean violence and discrimination. HCA's founders viewed the designation as part of a pattern of government-based discrimination that lacked medical justification. Even so, they could not simply deny that HIV/AIDS posed a threat to their community, as some had done. Exaggerated or otherwise, there were growing numbers of New Yorkers of Haitian origin who were becoming ill, and there were no visible efforts to protect or assist them. One HCA project coordinator expressed the founders' sense that they had to organize "for our people" because "no one else will."

In addition to violence and fear, public responses to the Haitian risk-group designation included economic discrimination and calls for harsher immigration restrictions (Farmer 1992, 212–14). The Haitian community, therefore, had to address AIDS in their midst on many levels. HCA provided information about HIV/AIDS to help the community fight the new source of discrimination without simply denying that there were Haitians dying from AIDS. They combined criticism of the popular race-based AIDS discourse with pragmatic programs for HIV/AIDS education and care. Much of their focus, however, remained on discrimination. Their defining public event would come in April 1990, when the Food and Drug Administration (FDA) imposed a ban on blood donation by Haitians. The agency coordinated a mass protest in New York's Times Square that drew an estimated fifty thousand marchers.

The Network

The fourth group ("it was a forum, not an organization"), the New York AIDS Network, focused its attention on treatment information. The Network brought together gay political and medical issues, introducing government epidemiologists to the community's own doctors. Participants included activists, gay men from the city who were just becoming mobilized, and medical practitioners affiliated with the St. Marks Community Clinic, a gay-oriented health clinic that, along with GMHC's clinic work, was the precursor of Community Health Project (CHP, later reorganized as the Callen-Lorde Community Health Center). Among their many functions, the Network provided an outlet for the latest medical information. They began meeting informally at the end of 1982, announcing their existence through an advertisement in *The Native* in February 1983. They worked with the CDC and against the city from the start; their campaigns were directed toward building a network between themselves and public health agencies. "Our premise was the legitimacy of the issue," a founding member explained. "What's happening? What can we do? Who can we contact?"

The Network fostered elite connections, including closeted gay political aides in New York City and Washington, D.C., who fed them the earliest possible information. As described by the same informant, "The tentacles of the network were amazing. We had friends on the inside." There was an "immense underground [of sympathetic gays] hidden everywhere." The Network collected data from doctors throughout the city and passed reliable statistics to the CDC. One informant indicated that it had taken the group "a while" to realize that the CDC actually wanted them to call and pass on their own data. They had initially viewed this as more of a pressure tactic, more to chide the researchers into action than to actually collaborate with them. It quickly became a form of street-level epidemiology, which informants perceived as a mechanism for keeping government researchers on the right track. "We called the CDC to tell them our numbers. They were a little behind. It started in the hundreds. I remember when we reached 1,000."

HEAL

Last, Health Education AIDS Liaison (HEAL) was, according to its 1995 mission statement, "founded in 1982 with the purpose of providing information, hope and support regarding natural ways of healing through alternative, holistic and non-toxic therapies." Informants there rephrased their goal as "disempowering the whitecoats," by which they referred not only to those who invoked medical authority over patient groups but to those who treated HIV/AIDS as a medical issue rather than a psycho-spiritual one and to those who fostered the "myth" that HIV caused AIDS. Opposed to all whose work defined "the AIDS zone," the mental-physical location where belief in one's own illness leads to symptoms of HIV/AIDS, HEAL necessarily did not foster close relations with state agencies. Although they were familiar with the work of treatment activists and buyers' clubs and were willing to work with them on alternative therapies, HEAL never formed a consistent working relationship with these organizations either. "They push us out," one member explained. A GMHC contact referred to HEAL as "an odd little niche" in the spectrum of community-based HIV/AIDS work. When HEAL refused to endorse any medical prophylactic process at all, many of the community-based help lines, which had referred clients to them for support needs, dropped them from the contact lists. HEAL, therefore, remained an isolate in the HIV/AIDS field and did not participate in the majority of the interactions examined in this study.

NETWORK ORIGINS

The first community-based organizational efforts were characterized by great uncertainty. The most significant fact about HIV/AIDS on which everyone could agree in 1981–1982 was that no one knew what it was. People died, and their doctors could not say what they had died of, if or how it was transmissible, or what one could do about it. There was no relevant expertise, and so community leaders began to create their own. The first organizations were either informal offshoots of existing organizations or regroupings of activists with a shared history. None began with a structure, a stated mission, or a name. Each started with the impression that it was working essentially alone, and four of the first five actively sought support from existing agencies in the domain of health and human services. As more information became available, and as the organizers gained experience, they discovered that they could get more help and better information from each other than from the state. Developing a greater sense of collective purpose, their efforts expanded into specialized tasks such as hotlines for people with AIDS, fundraisers for medical research, and community-based epidemiology. Central to each of these efforts was the need to generate, study, and disseminate any useful knowledge on the subject.

Almost as mysterious to those involved was the peculiar silence surrounding the emerging epidemic. With the exception of one or two articles in *The New York Native*, a gay newspaper, there had been virtually no media coverage of AIDS. Community organizers contrasted AIDS with prior health crises: Legionnaire's Disease and the Swine Flu scare. Each of these health threats had engendered a national mobilization and weeks of headlines with only a few deaths. By comparison, an accelerating pattern of deaths among young, recently healthy gay men did not rate. In response to this silence, much of the community-based work sought recognition of their plight and validation of their concerns.

Numerous factors contributed to the relative silence on HIV/AIDS early on. One was that research on sexuality of any form was discouraged during the Reagan administration. It was not an auspicious time to have a sexually transmitted disease. A second factor was the larger social stigma attached to all of the issues pertaining to HIV/AIDS, from homophobia to fear of death. In response to both of these impediments, the organized community sought to "normalize" the discourse on AIDS. A significant goal of much of the early organizing became, in the words of one informant, to "get AIDS on the screen." (The exception was HEAL, whose interests might be characterized as exactly the opposite, to convince people not to be taken in by AIDS mythologizing.)

While each of the new care and service organizations targeted their own communities for information and services, they all shared an interest in encouraging a more "mainstream" discussion. They sought an acknowledgment that their lives were at risk, validation that this was a crisis, and understanding that HIV/AIDS was a social problem, not a personal one. They mobilized volunteers, wrote articles, held rallies, and made phone calls. But neither the new CBOs nor the health crisis itself was treated as a legitimate social phenomenon at that time. After the first few years of HIV/AIDS in New York City, community organizing meant a small minority of people from within marginal, almost hidden populations exchanging information among themselves. Meetings of the Network were described by an informant, approvingly, as a "gossip hotline." Gossip was about as close to epidemiology as most people could get throughout much of 1982.

Emergent Collective Identities

Raising AIDS awareness posed a significant dilemma for all concerned. In later years, shared responsibility for HIV/AIDS in one's community would come to be called "owning the disease," predicated on the positive values of caring for one's own. But earlier on, no one wanted to own it. For the affected communities to step forward and say that AIDS really *was* a gay disease, or an African American disease, or a disease of drug users, would be a reaffirmation of the broader stigma that already tied their ascribed identities to this "contamination." As Joseph Gusfield (1981) has pointed out, accepting responsibility is easily confused with accepting blame. As long as the rest of the world was silent, those most affected had to take ownership of HIV/AIDS in their communities. Yet, as they took ownership, it allowed the rest of the world to remain silent.

Among the many community-based nonprofit organizations of the early 1980s, GMHC was the most self-conscious about defining the field of community work and their own location within it. They simultaneously propagated the messages that AIDS was a significant area for legitimate concern and that GMHC was a significant organization in the AIDS world. The group adopted the motto "First in the Fight against AIDS," with its multiple meanings. Eventually leaving research to the scientific community for the most part, GMHC came to define its primary mission around the delivery of uncensored information and daily-living assistance to people living with HIV/AIDS, whose needs they believed they understood better than anyone else.

Although it faced no explicit pressures to do so, GMHC established itself according to what its leaders perceived would win favor within the public health sector. "GMHC, originally a fairly innovative organization, was learning the ropes and would avoid political confrontations. Just eighteen months after its birth, at the U.S. Conference of Mayors in June 1983, GMHC impressed the participants with carefully presented documentation, including flowcharts and formal job descriptions, that, 'to [GMHC] President [Paul] Popham were the stuff of a sound organization'" (Perrow and Guillèn 1990, 109; quoting Shilts 1987, 325). One GMHC staff member identified 1984 as the time when GMHC moved from "street identity issues more firmly into service provision." They positioned themselves to take responsibility for their communities' service needs, not their political interests, in exchange for support from the public health sector.

Within its first few months, GMHC formed close connections with members of the Centers for Disease Control, the New York City Department of Health, and clinicians who were treating AIDS patients. In conjunction with the New York AIDS Network, which had close ties to city government and the state department of health, GMHC influenced the shape and mission of the state's AIDS Institute, founded in 1983. Community organizers helped to secure the appointment of former GMHC executive director Mel Rosen as the institute's first director.

GMHC chose its direction early on, defining types of work for which they would not take the lead, thereby defining empty spaces in the organizational field for others to occupy. They elected to follow a professional, social service model and to seek federal support. Several of the group's initial organizers had backgrounds and connections in social services and knew how to work profitably in this arena. In 1986, then-president Richard Dunne wrote that with their professional public image GMHC "has been very successful in getting funds allocated" (Dunne 1987, 155). Eight years later, a department head echoed the same sentiment: "Federal agencies love us. . . . Grantsmanship is what we're good at," adding that this necessarily precluded some amount of participatory democracy. "One doesn't run a multi-million dollar agency that way." Philip Kayal, a member who has written extensively about the organization, characterized "GMHC's ambiance" as "quite astounding, if not notorious, for a community-based organization. It is well-housed, professionally staffed, and remarkably well appointed" (1993, 109).

GMHC chose to avoid addressing any judgmental questions regarding sexual activity or expression, and they avoided political advocacy of any single "appropriate" policy. This meant that they could not take a stand on the safety of bathhouses and that they did not want to become involved in politics, even as others in the community organized protests and rallies on these very topics.[2] In their second newsletter in February of 1983, GMHC appealed to the gay community to adopt political abstinence when facing HIV/AIDS. "There is one thing we must not allow AIDS to become, and that is a *political* issue among ourselves. It's not. It's a health issue for us" (Kramer 1989, 27, quoting GMHC, emphasis in original). The target of this phase of their work was principally the gay community, particularly people with AIDS but also friends, family, and other affected people whom they recruited as volunteers, invited to education forums, and pressed for donations.

Although GMHC has been singled out for its participation in the bureaucracy of the public health service system (or, as one informant asked, "Why is there a dress code at an AIDS organization?"), they also participated in the less formal community support system. Organizers were aware of the potential limitations of that position, but they were hopeful that they would be taken seriously by policy makers. Later, an informant recalled, there would be "active debates . . . over institutionalism versus street activism." A different source said that they had struggled against becoming part of "the wallpaper" of the AIDS world. The group was committed to not being a social movement organization, but they knew that "both needed to be done."[3]

In contrast to GMHC's corporate style, the Network's meetings were attended by "anyone who knew something" about AIDS in New York. This included people from GMHC, the CDC, and the city Department of Health, although, according to one informant, "there were no 'members' in the network, and no 'representatives' from elsewhere." Meeting once every two weeks, they parsed through literally all available data from all sources and chose short-term follow-up tasks. Some items required some discussion, but few required a decision. The group did not take positions or plan events, as such. The Network maintained no long-term agenda and had no statement of purpose. The meetings were advertised and open to all, drawing up to twenty-five regulars and an equal number of occasional visitors.

Larry Kramer's history of the time differs a little from that of the current study's informants. The Network, he wrote, "was formed by many who felt left out of GMHC, which, unfortunately, was gaining an 'elitist' reputation. . . . It was to the AIDS Network that these veterans of years of involvement in the gay movement came, as well as newcomers who shared their desires for more aggressive tactics of confrontation" (Kramer 1989, 57).[4] There were certainly clashes between the two groups. Toward the end of its existence, the Network had considered reorganizing as an umbrella organization to coordinate among the growing number of new community groups. But, I was told, "the established organizations objected." Melinda Cuthbert's research found evidence for both realities. "Founders suggest that invitations were extended broadly and the membership remained open. Others argue that the organization was started by a select group of self-appointed leaders who were in key positions" (1990, 122). Leaders of the Network, apart from the clinicians, were also prominent in local gay organizations (Clifford 1992, 56–57). The group invited all kinds of newly involved people to attend and participate. Yet it was a networking forum for those who were already heavily involved, connected, and active. Informally, the Network connected the dots throughout the burgeoning HIV/AIDS field and between these organizations and the public health sector.

Although the main focus of the Network was research and treatment, the group also sought to influence the environment in which this work took place. Using its connections, the Network was able to pursue political goals of benefit to the entire community (which they perceived as having its center in New York's gay community), including securing support from the Koch administration for a Lesbian and Gay Community Services Center on 13th Street. The center became the new meeting space for the Network and the unofficial headquarters for AIDS concerns within the gay community. Once there, the composition of the meetings changed, as did the focus of the group. The group became larger and divided between two almost incompatible functions: continuing to operate loosely as "the newsletter of AIDS" and presenting formally organized public programs—education, colloquia, and discussions of issues. Connections with the health sector became more routinized as the Network helped to draft city confidentiality procedures, guidelines for protecting the blood supply, and nondiscrimination AIDS policies for city agencies, including the police and fire departments. When the New York State Department of Health set out to establish the AIDS Institute, the Network provided community representation.

Within a few years of the Network's founding, the group recognized that all of its concerns were being more formally pursued elsewhere by other CBOs. This had both positive and negative consequences. An informant stated, for example, that the Network had produced the first safer-sex campaign in the city, which, due to their independence, was "very explicit; GMHC could not distribute something like this back then." But for that reason, the group had become "the dumping ground for whatever issue the established groups couldn't dirty their hands with." The more "connected" the other organizations were, the less willing they were to pursue controversial agendas. The Network, as a looser affiliation of social actors without a formal mission, was tossed into every political storm. At the same time, their influence was being offset by the growth of the more specialized groups that the Network had helped to seed. In 1985, with most of its participants working in other CBOs and its mission divided among so many concentrated efforts, the New York AIDS Network voted to dissolve. General-purpose AIDS organizations were either giving way to emerging specialist groups or becoming more specialized themselves.

Over a period of less than four years, a new collective identity, "AIDS victim," came into being, was refined ("people affected by AIDS") and reimagined ("people living with HIV/AIDS"), and transformed into an organizing asset. The transformation of collective identity first followed and then led the public consciousness of the condition. AIDS had been initially identified as a "gay cancer," and then as a syndrome popularly and imprecisely attached to the "at-risk" communities. By 1984, it had not yet become known as a virus or even a medical condition in the normal sense of these things. It was spoken of as a threat, a stigma, and a plague. Members of the most affected communities divided. Some responded to the medical threat primarily and took ownership of the condition. Others responded more to the social stigma and the negative associations that are linked to blame and hostility. From the social perspective, it was useful to deny ownership. Thus, "HIV/AIDS" work emerged from the heart of an active, organized, and politically experienced gay community to quickly become its own field. Outside of the private circles of community organizers on the one hand and epidemiologists on the other, the origins, growth, and response to the new crisis were mostly unnoticed.

THE GROWTH OF THE AIDS COMMUNITY, 1984–1986

The earliest HIV/AIDS community-based organizations in New York City had all approached AIDS as a crisis of health and health care. They defined their own work in relation to the agencies of the public health sector. Even HEAL was merely alternative, not oppositional. From the first days and through the first years, the community-based mobilization in response to HIV/AIDS could have been incorporated into public, state-centered efforts. But there was not enough of a public framework for this to happen, and so they remained apart.

Once the groundwork had been laid, the active community had an organizational space in which to think about, discuss, and create the field of AIDS work. They sought information from the government and received little. They sought support and got less. Gradually, in this collective space, the organized community became self-supporting and self-generating. Rather than merely filling in until the health sector could get organized, the community sought to take control of HIV/AIDS work. One of the consistent themes that emerged during the interviews for this book was that the first wave of organizers had been waiting for the formal response to HIV/AIDS before they jumped in. Several informants for this study have indicated that they were aware of HIV/AIDS for years before volunteering anywhere, but they had assumed "it would be taken care of." Even after they started working on HIV/AIDS issues, they were still waiting. As one early volunteer, later a professional staff member at a different CBO, expressed it, "I kept thinking I would go back to being an actor."

Early network growth depended on the active community's realization that it was not being taken care of, that they could no longer wait. As the organizers and volunteers shifted their perspectives from temporary measures to long-term planning, their efforts moved from occasional informational or fundraising sessions to building stable infrastructures. As they began to recognize that they were not assisting the city or federal government but standing in for it, they began to develop more of an oppositional consciousness. This consciousness fostered the growth of an "AIDS community" discourse and significantly altered the course of community organizing.

By 1984, the epidemic had grown, but the political context remained essentially unchanged. Several new organizations had formed, and additional communities had mobilized. Health officials had settled on a name for AIDS—Acquired Immune Deficiency Syndrome—and several of the informally constituted community efforts incorporated as new CBOs with *AIDS* in their names. The major news media had published a few stories, though usually not the stories that the community would have wanted. For the organized community, the issue of the moment was marginalization. Community-building efforts began to converge on questions of exclusion and from there, recognition and empowerment. Communities began to claim ownership of HIV/AIDS.

HIV/AIDS itself was disdained. The proximate conditions associated with high rates of HIV/AIDS, including poverty, homosexuality, and drug use, were associated with further social marginalization. An unusual number of people with AIDS in the early 1980s had already lacked the support systems that they needed for even the simple tasks of daily living. Others, having become sick, subsequently lost their jobs and hence their insurance and often their homes as well. If they did not begin in poverty and seclusion, they often ended up there. This placed a tremendous burden of care and support on those community organizations that offered help to the sick.

AIDS volunteers in New York invented "the buddy system" in which young men and women signed on to visit people with AIDS, clean for them, do their shopping or dog walking, and bring them to and from medical appointments. In many cases, the buddies sat with the men as they died, and occasionally they arranged their funerals. In later years, as many more people with AIDS died at home with their families, AIDS orphans would become a new social problem, and elderly caregivers, usually grandmothers, would become responsible for them (Joslin 2002). But in the early 1980s, young adults in their twenties and thirties were presiding over the care and the deaths of others of their generation.

Daily Living

Gradually the new caregiving roles became a routine part of life within certain quarters of the city, and they became correspondingly more organized. Three innovative organizations—God's Love We Deliver (GLWD), the Momentum Project, and Bailey House—incorporated in 1985 to provide daily-living assistance to people with HIV/AIDS. GLWD began with two people in one apartment, following a period of volunteer work by the group's founder, Ganga Stone. Stone took on responsibility for a few people in late stages of HIV disease who were unable to care for themselves and scheduled their friends to bring them meals every day. Once organized, GLWD contacted local restaurants, many of them three- and four-star venues, and convinced them to donate food, which volunteers then delivered on foot and by bicycle to a growing list of homebound people with HIV/AIDS. Within its first year, GLWD mobilized hundreds of volunteers for relatively manageable, nonpolitical tasks. More significantly, they reached a different pool of people in New York who wanted to help do something in the face of HIV/AIDS but did not want to become activists or full-time volunteers. They also formed inroads into new areas of government support for community groups, ultimately gaining an eighty-thousand-dollar grant from New York State's Nutrition Assistance Program, the first of many such grants.

Organizers and caregivers identified new needs daily, and volunteers scrambled to fill the gaps. Pastoral organizations, such as the Momentum Project, opened additional food and clothing distribution sites specifically for people living with AIDS. The Momentum Project began in 1985 as a collaboration between GMHC's recreation program and St. Peter's Church in Harlem. Organized by Peter Avitabile, a GMHC volunteer, the group provided food, counseling (including both entitlements assistance and pastoral counseling), and a supportive place for poor and homeless people with AIDS to congregate. Momentum was defined around social service delivery to "underserved" populations. Momentum brought food to those who had no homes. They operated out of the poorest neighborhoods and sought out the least visible people living with HIV/AIDS. "The gay community is really on top of things," an informant explained. "Other groups were not; so we go there. . . . [The fact] that this population is not anyone's constituency is a real problem."

Despite vocal opposition from organizations of the religious right, which were politically ascendant during these years, church-based organizations in New York successfully mobilized new resources in support of the rising number of destitute HIV/AIDS patients. In 1985, ARC took over a renovated hotel building purchased by the city and began to construct Bailey House to provide temporary safe housing for homeless people with HIV/AIDS. (Years later, ARC reorganized under the name Bailey House. They currently operate three houses mostly funded by New York City.) Approved by the city only to develop a shelter for homeless people living with HIV/AIDS, Bailey House instead created a full-time subsidized residence. According to Cuthbert's informants, "the City wanted Bailey House to be a shelter, but shelter residents are not considered to have addresses, so they are not eligible for welfare or SSI" (1990, 147). Bailey House gave residents a permanent address and helped them to navigate the city's complex social service entitlements procedures.

Empowerment as a Movement

The empowerment movement for people with HIV/AIDS grew directly out of the intersection of these social support efforts and the cultural and identity work ongoing among gay activists. The landmark event of this movement was the Second National AIDS Forum in 1983 in Denver, Colorado, sponsored by the National Gay and Lesbian Health Education Foundation. The 1983 Denver meeting produced a declaration of the rights of PWAs, including "the right to die — and LIVE — in dignity" (emphasis in original).[5] The Denver Principles, as the document became known, introduced the now common phrase "people with AIDS" in an effort to replace the more marginalizing "AIDS victims." The term, and its later incarnation, "people living with HIV," stressed people rather than transmission rates and living rather than dying. And while the Denver conference was particularly a lesbian and gay event, the declaration explicitly sought to speak for all those seeking new ways to live in the face of HIV, "officially" separating AIDS activism from gay activism. The Denver Principles became the founding statement of the empowerment movement for people living with HIV/AIDS.

The empowerment movement took several directions. First, through new member/client CBOs such as the People with AIDS Coalition (PWAC, later PWAC/NY), people with HIV/AIDS created spaces in which to provide mutual support, information exchange, and advocacy, guided by their own needs and experiences. A PWAC/NY informant, explaining the group's philosophy, defined it as "a safe place for people to come in and deal with their issues." A former PWAC staff member, later working at the Community Health Project, recalled the PWAC experience as particularly "compelling. . . . It was very exciting to see people taking charge of what was going on with them and not be victimized by it." These personal support efforts also fostered connections among therapeutic communities, developing AIDS support groups through agencies like the Manhattan Center for Living and later, AIDS therapy groups at Friends in Deed (FID, an offshoot of the Manhattan Center).

The support organizations encouraged people with HIV/AIDS to plan for their lives and to take charge of their treatments, which helped to generate an aggressive patient advocacy movement. The movement, according to a PWAC/NY source, was "unique because we listen to what [health authorities] say and use it in our newsletters." But the empowerment movement was also premised on an active distrust of the motives of state agents. For many newsletter readers, the clinical data produced by the National Institutes of Health wasn't validated until it passed the community-based review represented by PWAC publication.

The community and the relevant government agencies at the local and state level were both collaborators and antagonists through this period of expansion. One reason for the growth of new community-based organizations was that the formal policies of city and state government did not prioritize HIV/AIDS or even always recognize it. Yet, for this very reason, the relevant agencies needed to support the community efforts. They simply had to keep much of this support indirect or even hidden. As a result, community organizers often perceived city and state agencies as obstacles to be overcome rather than as allies. Importantly, however, the agencies involved did not actually oppose or significantly interfere with the community's growth.

The community groups that were moving from information redistribution to care, therapy, daily-living assistance, and even medical referrals were thereby moving out of the territory of private charity and self-help and into the traditional domains of the welfare state. The city, which had very few comparable services of its own and which was perpetually struggling with an overburdened public health care system, quietly encouraged this development. The New York State Department of Health also provided new money for qualified AIDS service organizations. Both city and state health officials helped community groups become "qualified" through both formal and informal assistance. When the Network and others sought city support to open the Lesbian and Gay Community Services Center, the Koch administration required them to provide a community-based health clinic there as well. A new group, the Community Health Project, described below, provided this service. A CHP informant described the relationship between the group and the city as he had perceived it: "I think because the city never wanted to take care of our community, so if someone else was willing to, that was good enough for them. And we were certainly providing a public service because otherwise all these patients would be dumped into the public health system."

The state had been active in research and epidemiology but had not sought the few contacts they had among the affected communities and didn't always know what to do with them once they had been established. "Leaving the male gay community to respond to the AIDS crisis meant that the state with all its resources was allowed to take a distancing role, emphasizing coordination rather than direct service when it finally did have to act" (Perrow and Guillén 1990, 83). The organized community, by taking charge of HIV/AIDS work, claimed authority over the issue, even ahead of the state, which had lost some of its legitimacy in their eyes. One activist stated that in the 1980s "there was a sense of community again . . . based very much on the understanding that the government was not going to do it for us." Community-based AIDS work, having become the official conduit for all state expenditures for AIDS care, acquired a higher degree of legitimacy within the public health sector. Meanwhile, the state's dependence on the care and information network that the community had built "as a result of the government failure to do so in the early years further supported the development of this alternative infrastructure" (Cuthbert 1990, 41). At the city level, government agencies and community organizations served each other's interests and needs with a reserve that often looked like hostility.

Long-Term Planning

The community-based infrastructure, particularly through the patients' empowerment movement, fostered the growth of a new organizational form: buyers' clubs. Buyers' clubs collated research on possible treatments, debunking some, accepting others with side-effect warnings, and publishing fact sheets and newsletters to those seeking information and options. While the already-existing alternative treatments movement taught people living with HIV/AIDS about such modalities as visualizations, meditation, herbs, and crystals, the buyers' clubs concentrated on gaining access to forms of treatment not approved by the Food and Drug Administration. They purchased, smuggled, or manufactured potential treatments, particularly antibiotics, from all over the world and distributed them at cost to their many members. Prior to the general availability of AZT in 1987 and continuing after, advocates of alternative treatments had collected and even investigated anecdotal reports of the efficacy of aspirin, egg lipids, acupuncture, extracts from the bark of Japanese trees, pastes made from exotic fungi, and any other possible substance or therapy (including drinking one's own urine) that anyone had used to fight opportunistic infections, strengthen the immune system, or combat the symptoms of HIV/AIDS. The buyers' clubs treated alternative therapies and FDA-approved drugs equally, providing fact sheets and warnings for both and sending patients back to their doctors armed with specific questions about drug interactions, resistance, and mortality rates. They also arranged to acquire the leftover prescription drugs from the estates of those who died, distributing the prohibitively expensive drugs cheaply to their members. Perhaps most importantly, given their interest in treatment evaluation, the clubs provided regular meeting spaces to exchange case histories among their members, performing their own versions of reliability measures and adding to the knowledge base of the "treatment community."

The clubs operated on the fringes of the law, working somewhat as consumer advocates and somewhat as smugglers. Buyers' clubs represented a new degree of illegitimate community organizing, a break with the pursuit of institutional acceptance and a greater commitment to community ownership of HIV/AIDS. They called themselves "the AIDS underground." The first and largest formally recognized buyers' club, the PWA Health Group, was created in 1986 (incorporated 1987) by Michael Callen (with Joe Sonnabend and Thomas Hannan), "out of the approval of AZT." (AZT was the first approved drug therapy for AIDS, but it was toxic in high doses and was not highly effective. The Health Group wanted something better.) One organizer described the group as "the most official, most conservative face of" the AIDS underground. Even so, for its first few years, the PWA Health Group "worked out of a church so the police would not bust down the doors."

While the PWA Health Group specialized in the obscurities of clinical trials and standards of regulation, a later group, Direct AIDS Alternative Information Resources (DAAIR), combined access to drugs in trials with the potential benefits of hundreds of herbal remedies. One Health Group informant stated that they had a "complementary relationship to DAAIR," but DAAIR sometimes perceived them "as a threat." Fred Bingham, founder and director of DAAIR, described his organization as part buyers' club, part alternative treatment study group, and part information clearinghouse. Informants at both organizations characterized themselves as much more closely aligned to each other than either was to HEAL, the alternative therapy CBO that one long-time buyers' club participant dismissed as a "hypnosis group." Yet the three organizations' forms and practices resembled one another more than any of them resembled the rest of the field. HEAL, although isolated from most interorganizational processes, expressed empathy toward the buyers' clubs.

"The most radical stuff is the underground drug network," one informant offered, as an expression of respect. In 2000, DAAIR merged with the PWA Health Group.

By the end of 1986, as part of what one counselor at Body Positive called "the maturing of the field of AIDS," those involved with HIV/AIDS empowerment became attentive to the fact that an increasing number of HIV-positive people did not have AIDS. "So there was a population who were not on their death beds." Setting off what would become a wave of new organizational initiatives throughout 1987, Michael Hirsch and others at the People with AIDS Coalition formed Body Positive, whose mission was "to teach people how to live" with HIV. This was not a function that others were pursuing. As one activist associated with Body Positive observed, "There is and will be an increasing need to deal with people who don't do the convenient thing and die." The reference was to the public health sector's lack of preparedness for the long-term-care needs of HIV-positive individuals, whose well-being was left to their private communities of care.

In both positive and negative ways, HIV/AIDS was finally becoming normal and losing its sense of crisis, and community workers were beginning to see HIV/AIDS involvement as their new careers, not as a diversion from their careers. As one informant at PWAC explained about the group's change in direction, "My hope when I started was to be unemployed." Drawing together support groups, treatment information, peer education, and empowerment, Body Positive began the process of helping people with HIV readjust their lives for the long haul. Among other services, the organization published a resource guide for living with HIV/AIDS in New York City. Like the empowerment organizations from which it grew, Body Positive sought to develop the expertise of the patient community. They linked experts to the newly diagnosed, and connected isolated individuals with the support network of New York CBOs.

State-Community Relations in the First and Second Waves

The early risers of HIV/AIDS organizing had established the terms of the discussion, for those who wished to have a discussion, and established models of collective organizing for mutual aid and self-protection. The two crises that arose together, starting in 1981, were that people were becoming sick or were dying from HIV/AIDS and that there was no public recognition of it. The initial organizations needed to address the medical and social issues together. They sought to convince anyone and everyone that there was a crisis, that something had to be done, and that they could help. By 1983, a visible field of organizations had begun to take shape and grow.

Within this emerging field, there was a constant movement of people and information and a shared sense of purpose. The mission was "AIDS" in the most general and comprehensive sense. Mostly made up of volunteers, the organized field worked within the affected communities to help in any way they could and outside the communities to generate visibility—to make AIDS real. Deliberate alarmists, like Larry Kramer, sought to portray the worst-case scenario in order to create awareness among their communities and spur public agencies to action. Many of these scenarios have come true, with more than 120,000 cases of AIDS in New York City confirmed by the end of 2004 and an additional 26,000 living with HIV (Bureau of AIDS Epidemiology 2005).

After a period of silence, the fear kicked in. Occasional newspaper coverage of "risk groups" defined unpopular subpopulations (gay men, Black immigrants, etc.) as dangerous people. After too many premature deaths, gay men and others in affected communities moved quickly from ignorance to concern to panic. The next groups to emerge, therefore, were less concerned to organize volunteers on behalf of people with HIV/AIDS and more concerned to organize people living with HIV/AIDS to work for themselves. These newer groups, which focused on health, medicines, safe living spaces, and emotional support, entered into an existing field and networked with the groups that were already there.

State-community relations were confused and inconsistent from the start. The earliest groups had mostly assumed that government agencies would take the lead in the response to HIV/AIDS. Some of the early organizers, particularly those with experience in the social services, spoke of shock or disillusion when this did not occur. Others, notably including Larry Kramer (1983, 1989) and Vito Russo (1988), who viewed the issue through the lens of gay politics, accused the state of deliberately allowing HIV/AIDS to spread. At the same time, most of the new organizations were able to get some money and other forms of support from state and city agencies some of the time.

The first-wave organizations provided the impetus and the direction behind several of the most important and lasting responses to HIV/AIDS adopted at the city and state levels. The first was the founding of the Center in 1983, with the active participation and support of the city. Currently known as the Lesbian, Gay, Bisexual & Transgender Community Center, the Center has flourished. At one point in the early 1990s, the Center was hosting regular meetings for more than three hundred groups, including many of the HIV/AIDS CBOs in this study.

The AIDS Institute was the second major institution through which the community stamp was imprinted into state policy and practice. The institute itself was created and funded by the New York State Department of Health but was designed and administered, to a large degree, by community leaders. As noted above, the AIDS Institute's first director came from GMHC. In 1984, the AIDS Institute began funding much of GMHC's case management work through its new Community Service Program (CSP). As the CSP grew, numerous other community groups were funded to perform similar services following "the GMHC model."

The second wave of organizing, working with a greater sense of community ownership, fewer expectations about the state, and more informal inroads into government, established a kind of limited partnership among different agencies. Defining HIV/AIDS work as something that belonged in the private nonprofit sector, rather than as a strictly public problem, seems to have facilitated communication and collaboration between the two sectors.

The nonprofit community-based organizations actively networked with each other from the start. Connections throughout the field grew denser as the field grew. The first groups provided resources to the emerging groups, such as knowledge, contacts, and material support. The missions of the second-wave groups were defined with reference to the first wave. GMHC had a hotline, and HCA and ARC had information hotlines and other forms of outreach to the newly diagnosed. Volunteers and other participants quickly determined which services and support activities were most needed but not yet provided. The second-wave organizations provided those functions, while the first-wave groups referred clients. Many of the staff and volunteers in the newer groups came out of the initial organizations, and connections between them were often tight. One early volunteer, who worked for several agencies before becoming a professional service provider at a government-sponsored agency, recalled that "there was very little duplication. No one was doing what Ganga [Stone of GLWD] was doing. No one was doing what GMHC was doing [or] what PWAC was doing." Describing the movement of individual staff and volunteers around all of the different groups in those days, he called it "an incestuous community."

The organized community was larger, farther reaching, and tight. The groups had finally achieved much of the recognition they had sought—for themselves, their communities, and the seriousness of their cause. Their efforts were not comprehensive, however. Some groups, and hence some perspectives on HIV/AIDS priorities, were far more visible than others. The tight bonds between organizations also meant that interorganizational practices were becoming standardized, and new participants had less opportunity to influence the nature of those practices. There were gaps within the new community space, mostly defined along the traditional boundaries of race, class, and gender. Chapters 3 and 4 will address some of the new organizing efforts that arose to fill these spaces.

NOTES

1. The Judson Memorial Church remains a central venue in the world of HIV/AIDS in New York and has been the site of many events, speeches, and gatherings. In 1992, for example, on the day before election day, the political funeral of Mark Lowe Fisher wound from the church at Washington Square to the Republican National Headquarters on 43rd Street. (See "Political Funerals" at www.actupny.org/diva/polfunsyn.html.)

2. Gay bathhouses were popular social venues in the 1980s in cities with large, open gay populations. They included stage shows and other entertainments as well as the opportunities for men to meet and have sex in the bathhouse itself.

3. An ACT UP (AIDS Coalition to Unleash Power) informant used this precise phrase during an interview, but several sources from GMHC and other groups have used almost exactly the same wording.

4. The New York AIDS Network certainly did adopt a more confrontational stance, particularly with regard to the Koch administration. However, Kramer's historical version must be read cautiously, as he himself describes this period as the start of his losing battle with GMHC over the question of "more aggressive tactics of confrontation." As the Network was more receptive to this attitude, it is likely that some activists did go there, as Kramer suggests, out of dissatisfaction with GMHC's integrative policies.

5. An informant at PWAC has suggested that the Denver Principles were consciously fashioned on the model of the Seneca Falls Convention of 1848, from which had come the Declaration of Sentiments linking women's rights to the ideal of citizenship, though it is not clear if this connection was widely discussed.

Chapter Three

Collective Identity and Reorganization

In 1985, the Council of Churches for the City of New York asked Suki Ports to organize a conference on "AIDS in the minority community." Ports recalled how she had first sought support from the city and other local funders. "They said 'why would you want that? AIDS is not a minority issue.' So we went to the CDC and the big service organizations that had all this money, and they said 'why would you want that? AIDS is not a minority issue.'"

The initial wave of mobilizing in response to HIV/AIDS in New York created a collective identity and defined an organizational space around it. The boundaries of the space were broadly drawn, but much of the activity clustered tightly around gay male issues. The second wave of organizing greatly diversified the kinds of activities that were occurring within the most active clusters. From personal empowerment to media outreach, these groups reached out to a wider population of potential participants, linking newly diagnosed individuals to networks of care and knowledge.

The third wave of organizing was driven by those who did not have a discernible location in the existing organizational space. Drawing on the resources of *both* public and private sources, in and out of the field, they expanded the definitions of what the field was. This definitional work targeted both public and private actors equally. In this way, they significantly altered the configuration of state-community relations. Defining their own needs and goals, the newer organizers operated with different expectations about who would support them and how. They drew upon the accomplishments and resources of the existing field while also working against the assumptions underlying the field's collective process.

EMPTY SPACES

Before researchers, the media, and the public had accepted that HIV would become a universal phenomenon, demographic reports demonstrated the degree to which the language of "risk groups" had become a source of confusion and difficulty for epidemiology and a powerful stigma for those to whom the label was applied. A Centers for Disease Control and Prevention (CDC) summary report for 1983 had indicated increasing incidence rates from around the nation, the majority identified with "the high risk groups previously described" (CDC 1983b). Even so, the report referred several times to cases of unidentified origin among patients who "denied belonging to known AIDS risk groups." Such patient self-reports did not undermine confidence in the risk-group model, however, as researchers noted that "the accuracy of data concerning sexual activity and IV drug use cannot be verified" (CDC 1983b). Despite conflicting data, both ownership of and culpability for HIV/AIDS had been fixed on a particular set of people, and they would not be easily shaken loose.

One difficulty with this model was that it created pockets of mystery as more and more cases fell outside its borders. Increasing numbers of the unidentified cases were among women, most of whom were assumed to be either injecting drug users or sexual partners of high-risk men, and were therefore explained, if not investigated, verified, or understood. As Mark Donovan observed, "The incongruities between non-gay, non-injecting drug using PWAs and prevailing stereotypes did not, however, lead to a reassessment of the negative constructions of gays and IDUs with AIDS, but instead led to the creation of new, identifiable groups of PWAs such as 'women with AIDS' and 'children with AIDS'" (1997, 123). They were, in a sense, risk groups of no known risk.

From this perspective, those in the newer demographic categories saw history repeat itself, up to a point. The public health sector had begun to adjust to HIV/AIDS but had not yet recognized the need to do anything for those who were both at risk and without resources. Yet, now that there was a public response to HIV/AIDS, the newer community groups were not as thoroughly rebuffed in their efforts to follow a more traditional "resource mobilization" model (McCarthy and Zald 1977), connecting their constituencies to HIV/AIDS agencies in both the public and the private sectors. Across demographic categories, their organizing efforts were often disjointed, related to one another only through their ties to the established field, or related through the efforts of the department of health.

"THE REST OF THE AIDS COMMUNITY"

Norms and values are locally constituted, as Emile Durkheim (1964) observed. Even in the social margins, some groups are less equal than others. "In New York City the political influence of homosexuals has not been impressive," Ron Aran and David Rogers (1990, 116) noted. But "other groups with high rates of HIV infection, such as IV drug users, prison inmates, and the homeless, fared even more poorly." Volunteerism across constituencies helped to spread the awareness of the range of HIV/AIDS issues throughout the active communities, but it never leveled the field (Cohen 1999). And it was not lost on members of those other groups that the image of HIV/AIDS that GMHC (Gay Men's Health Crisis) was successfully marketing did not look like them.

Organizers began to launch new groups targeting or serving people of color and other "underrepresented" communities in the mid-1980s. They worked with or grew out of the prior groups, but they did not ever seem to achieve parity with them in political, cultural, or economic terms. The most successful self-starting groups, with their professional public personas, had been highly influential in setting the agenda for service and care in their own images. Both their visibility and their imagery increased the likelihood that they would be commissioned to participate in the delivery of those services, particularly at the city level. The professionalism of the service community-based organizations (CBOs) aligned them with the public health system, and money was allocated according to their priorities. But their success created a rift between them and the more radical arms of the community, including the newer groups that were seeking political and legal change. Some suggested that the unequal distribution of funding reflected far more than the "White" groups' indigenous ability to mobilize limited resources (*Poz Magazine* 1997), proposing instead that they were becoming complicit in the enduring prejudices that kept HIV issues hidden from the public view. State and city agencies, meanwhile, had become comfortable helping the nonthreatening GMHC and its offshoots to provide basic services and education, while "the [injecting drug users] and the gay men and bisexuals in the minority community were virtually ignored" (Perrow and Guillén 1990, 83).

A wide range of social, political, and economic factors combined to make gay White men the face of HIV/AIDS in New York City. African American communities, already caught up in the politics and the stigmas of poverty and drug use, were "reluctant to 'own' the AIDS epidemic" (Dalton 1989, 205). For African American leaders to have embraced the "risk group" label would have conflicted with community empowerment efforts in the political realm.

Some have spoken of not wanting to confirm White prejudices about drug users in the African American community (Cohen 1999, 74). And where activists for gay rights had something to gain by openly discussing their sexual identities and behaviors, African American activists did not. The situation was similar for Latino communities, where discourse on sexual identity has been associated with "the domain of the secret and the forbidden" (Diaz 1997, 235). Meanwhile, among the state-funded, gay-centered, mostly White service organizations, "experienced activists . . . found that AIDS has turned them into professionals" (Altman 1988, 310). Successful inclusion in the world of social service provision and government grants drew the largest and oldest community-based organizations away from "the community." Or, as one minority activist explained, "GMHC has lost its *C*."

The marginalization of communities of color and the greater affinity that researchers and policy makers felt with the professional social service model of the mainstream organizations created a further difficulty for groups seeking to define a non-White HIV/AIDS agenda. African American and Latino issues were often perceived and discussed in terms of what made them "different," that is, unique to people of color. Heterosexually transmitted HIV, transfusion, and perinatal transmission were becoming old news and had been presented in the media from time to time as hazards to the "general population," with accompanying photographs of White women and children. Stories concerning communities of color with HIV/AIDS focused on drug users, their "deceived" sexual partners, and their "innocent" children (Cohen 1999, 177). Public and media sympathy with the innocent victims of the epidemic necessarily implied that the guilty ones were still out there, walking threats to public health and safety. In some cases, the media discourse was explicit in placing the blame for HIV/AIDS outside the boundaries of White culture. Mainstream press coverage exhibited a fascination with the quest for the origins of HIV, a quest that frequently involved African monkeys or Haitian "voodoo" (Cohen 1999, 173–75; Farmer 1992). The apparent comfort with which mainstream HIV/AIDS service organizations had begun to negotiate the HIV policy domain, combined with the black-and-white simplicity of the mass media's language of culpability (Hallett and Cannella 1994), kept issues of drugs, poverty, and access to health care off the agenda. Even in cases where the mainstream groups expanded their mandates, their "authority" depreciated the value or relevance of culturally specific knowledge or experience, leaving many with the feeling that they had been forced out of the discussion of their own lives. As Cathy Cohen (1999, 115) explained,

> This tension is heightened by what is perceived to be the disjunction or inconsistency between the staffing patterns of many white AIDS organizations, whose

staff members are primarily white men and lesbians, and the public, almost preachy stances they take on issues such as needle exchange, condom distribution in the high schools, and the development of an AIDS curriculum—issues that black AIDS activists lament are experienced most severely in communities of color.

Within the politically active gay organizations, homosexuality could be an identity claim that guided their outreach and their styles of presentation. It said little, initially, to gay people of color, and it was not particularly clear about the place of lesbians in the response to HIV/AIDS, let alone of straight women. African American homosexual men therefore almost had to choose between being gay *or* being Black when making contact with HIV/AIDS CBOs. African American women did not necessarily have either of those options. As a result of the relative neglect of people of color among gay HIV/AIDS organizations, the disinterest in lesbians and gay men within African American organizations, and popular media representations of HIV among African Americans as a problem exclusive to drug users (Peterson 1997), African American HIV/AIDS organizing had no clear identity or mandate. "The identity movements following from the CDC's definition has been very influential in AIDS," a community worker stated, "and very harmful."

The risk-group model had epidemiological value, but its use outside of research placed members of the identified groups at risk for all manner of threats and sanctions from a frightened public. The addition of "Haitian" to the list of risk populations, for example, directly triggered attacks on Caribbean New Yorkers. Subsequent immigration restrictions related to this classification exacerbated the tension between the Haitian community and the public health sector, culminating in the 1990 decision by the Food and Drug Administration (FDA) barring Haitians from donating blood (Farmer 1992, 218). In an editorial note in 1983, almost a year after the original classification, the CDC justified the scientific basis and appropriate use of risk-group identification, despite awareness that it had already "been used unfairly as a basis for social and economic discrimination" (CDC 1983a). Medical journals, the popular press, and "a variety of other scholarly journals" had run speculative articles about the Haitian origins of AIDS (Farmer 1992, 212). And while research continued to fail to support this thesis, and despite the fact that the CDC quietly dropped the Haitian risk designation in 1984 (a designation that had originally been based on only thirty-four cases [CDC 1982]), the popular confusion about Haitian culpability remained. The image and the associated speculation were sufficiently credible for the *Journal of the American Medical Association* to suggest, in 1986, that the presumed high rates of AIDS among Haitians were driven by the drinking of blood during "voodooistic rituals," among other absurdities (Farmer 1992, 3). By that time, health sector credibility among Haitians, and among many other communities of color, had plummeted.

Ernest Quimby (1993) summarized four "fundamental barriers" that limited the African American mobilization against HIV/AIDS during the 1980s. The first was "competing priorities," which referred to the existing strain on the resources of Black communities seeking to mobilize support for economic development and health care, and against discrimination and violence, among other issues. "Internal differences" among community leaders over the appropriate stance to take on AIDS, drugs, and homosexuality further impeded collective action. Many African Americans also viewed HIV/AIDS advocates in and out of the public health sector with "suspicion and skepticism." As Harlon Dalton expressed it, "The deep-seated suspicion and mistrust many of us feel whenever whites express a sudden interest in our well-being hampers our progress in dealing with AIDS" (Dalton 1989, 211). HIV prevention efforts such as syringe exchange were perceived to be poor substitutes for real solutions, including drug treatment, and as being forced on the Black community by White health officials (and White activists). Finally, the historical "lack of community-based education and prevention" meant that state-based service providers had little culturally useful knowledge about African Americans, while people in the communities had little basis on which to judge the merits of the attention they were receiving. Even after community organizing began, the gay-centered African American groups at the forefront of HIV/AIDS work were generally unable to create lasting connections to existing political and social organizations in the Black community (Quimby 1993, 220).

Comparable issues influenced the prospects for Latino organizing. As both gay and Latino organizations began to address the complex cultural milieu of Latino sexual behavior, they found it difficult to identify or address their target populations. Researchers and HIV/AIDS prevention workers introduced the term "men who have sex with men" to cover sexual acts among men who do not define themselves as homosexual. This term was intended to speak to, among others, young, mostly heterosexual Latino men who engaged in sexual acts with men, sometimes anonymously and generally outside of the structure of a defined relationship. To a large degree, the language recognized that not everyone conceptualized gender relations in simple binary terms of hetero/homo. At the same time, use of the term contributed to the idea that there are no gay Latinos. It has therefore been described as "deeply insensitive, insulting, and ultimately conspir[ing] with the homophobic silence that creates so much disruption, suffering and risky behavior" in the lives of gay Latino men (Diaz 1997, 7).

Organizing as a collective or a community requires, at the very least, a name or description around which to organize. The popularly held designations for HIV/AIDS risk groups and the exaggerated sense of boundaries between them left little room for people of color to self-organize. Thrown together as "minorities," however, or as "the rest of the AIDS community," as expressed by one Latino informant, the affected communities of people who didn't fit in the existing framework were able generate a wave of new activity. Their activities further altered, and in surprising ways may have improved, the dynamics of state-community relations.

Liminal Identity Categories, 1985–1988

Despite the early lack of institutional support for the Council of Churches' conference, organizer Suki Ports was able to draw together a small group of minority activists and professionals to help her secure funding. Originally intended to educate service providers, prevention educators, and health policy planners on the specific concerns of people of color outside of the mainstream service system, the conference served instead to "prove that this was an issue," and to create a working group to define the appropriate response. From this effort, the Minority Task Force on AIDS (MTFA) was created, with Ports as its first director.

The conference planners sought data from both the City Department of Health and the CDC on the incidence of HIV/AIDS among different ethnic groups, but neither agency had such data at that level of detail. The Department of Health was mostly working with a risk-group model in which most cases were either gay or drug related. Within that, they counted ethnic data as Black, White, Latino, or "other," and they were not aware of any cases among Asian Americans (Eckholdt et al. 1997). This, in turn, made it almost impossible to mobilize Asian and other groups, since the government had essentially declared them not to be at risk. As Nancy Stoller found in her study of HIV/AIDS organizing in San Francisco, "the development of Asian-American responses to the HIV/AIDS epidemic has been a struggle for visibility and particularity within an epidemic in which Asians and Pacific Islanders were first invisible and then seen as monocultural by dominant institutions" (Stoller 1998, 63). This conference thereby also provided the groundwork for efforts that would later become APICHA, the Asian and Pacific Islander Coalition on HIV and AIDS (Eckholdt et al. 1997).

MTFA opened its offices in Harlem and provided a combination of advocacy and services. Although they received more than enough requests for service, their community-building efforts were limited by widespread denial and fear. "We couldn't tell people what we were doing," Ports recalled. The group's offices did not display their name. Organizers felt that neither their presence nor their clients would have been tolerated in that neighborhood if anything of theirs had said "AIDS." The main office was a service center. For advocacy purposes, MTFA brought together a separate coalition of groups from different cities to form NMAC, the National Minority AIDS Council.

Around the same time, other CBOs took on responsibility for organizing among Latinos/Latinas, separate from the rest of the organized AIDS community. The Hispanic AIDS Forum (HAF) began work in 1985. HAF, which focused on services for "hard to reach populations" (Hispanic AIDS Forum n.d.), began as a small education and referral service managed by health and human service professionals, with a bilingual AIDS hotline run out of the offices of the Association of Puerto Rican Executive Directors. Its later service expansions included women's programs in the Bronx and Harlem and Spanish-language programs for gay and bisexual men (Elbaz 1992, 54).

HAF began with the assumption that neither the mainstream media nor the public health sector was going to reach out to Latino communities in response to the AIDS epidemic. Rather, both potential information sources had begun to impugn Latinos as "AIDS junkies" and other such neologisms that blamed drug users for the crisis and for the "crossover" of HIV into the heterosexual world. Given the public hostility, the difficulty of discussing sexual practices in public in Latino communities, and the defensiveness among Latino activists concerning the association of their communities with drug use, the prospects for meaningful and helpful AIDS education were not promising. Many Latinos eschewed the established AIDS service organizations, such as GMHC, where the literature and the education were most often directed to an openly gay audience. Even the relatively small amount of literature that was translated into Spanish did not speak to the experiences of the Latino community with sex or drugs. HAF, therefore, created a fairly small new forum in which to strategize a Latino-centered approach to HIV/AIDS prevention.

The Latino Coalition on AIDS (LCOA), which held its first "founding summit" in 1990, described their work as a combination of empowerment and education, but not service provision. That is, they addressed the needs of an entire community of affected people in political and cultural domains, through education, representation, and research, and through the support of programs of concern to their constituency. Fundamentally, the organization sought to make itself an authoritative source on HIV/AIDS issues in place of both health officials and traditional sources of community leadership. "These are people you're taught to respect in the Latino community: your mother, the priest, the teacher, the elderly, and your doctor," an LCOA outreach worker explained. That made the group's work particularly difficult, since it challenged all of those people. This informant described LCOA's mission, to bring culturally useful HIV/AIDS awareness to the Latino community in relation to comparable groups with different target populations. "Life Force does this for women; Housing Works does it for homeless people with HIV." LCOA also drew upon the experiences of ADAPT (the Association for Drug Abuse Prevention and Treatment), where some of the leadership of LCOA had previously worked. (ADAPT is discussed in chapter 4.)

Collectively, these groups formed a separate niche of community-based HIV/AIDS organizing. They consciously drew upon the opportunities and resources provided by the earlier groups while defining their mandates in contrast to the work already being done. An informant at the Latino Commission suggested that, unlike GMHC or Bailey House, LCOA was best at coordinating work from outside the health and social services sector. Their particular form of advocacy involved raising questions that others weren't asking, preferably in a public forum where their interests could influence others' agendas. Interesting to note, the other groups were often happy to follow their lead. "Because we don't provide services and such, we're not seen as a competitor, so we can do that." LCOA cosponsored educational symposia, gave awards to leaders in the field whose work impacted Latino health, and generally negotiated a complex exchange of legitimacy signs with health officials, researchers, and other CBOs.

The Latino HIV/AIDS organizations of this period needed to define their work as different, but not too different, from the core of the existing field of work. They remained somewhat apart from both the earlier and the later waves of "White" CBOs. They were rarely activists, but they worked with activists. They critiqued service providers for becoming too corporate, for serving majority community needs, and for favoring patients with better insurance. Yet Latino community organizing was, if anything, more dependent on public funding than most of the older groups, a fact that affected their organizational missions. Explaining why LCOA can get grants for drug counseling but not for health education, for example, a staff member observed, "You don't see a lot of Latino organizations getting funding to do work outside of what is seen as 'their specialty.'"

The public health sector's perceived tendency to lump all minority communities together as a single entity with a single set of needs created pressures on the Latino groups to cautiously coordinate. HAF, for example, which had remained relatively small for a number of years, had difficulty proving to funders that it could manage city or state grants on its own. Government funders disdained the smaller minority CBOs as "isolated organizations" that lacked backing by other community groups (Cuthbert 1990, 207). At the same time, MTFA, the most broadly directed minority CBO in existence during this period, had difficulty demonstrating to funders that they were sufficiently unique. MTFA was pressured to collaborate with groups like HAF on the grounds that it would be redundant to have both groups providing services to "the same" communities.

Previous studies on the development of HIV/AIDS community organizations in New York have stressed the importance of new funding streams to the expansion of education, awareness, prevention, and empowerment. None of the CBOs created by and for women nor those created by and for people of color were able to duplicate the considerable mobilization of resources that the mostly gay, mostly White, mostly male organizations had accomplished in pioneering the HIV/AIDS field. Unlike GMHC, PWAC (the People with AIDS Coalition), and the Momentum Project, organizations serving populations that lacked ownership of HIV/AIDS—such as women's groups and Latino organizations—"had embryonic existence until they obtained public funding" (Chambré 1997, 475).

By presenting themselves as fulfilling a recognized public mission, but for an underserved community, Latino organizations were able to justify in a derivative fashion their right to exist and to receive public support. These organizations thereby created an institutionally backed home for work on HIV/AIDS in Latino communities. Volunteers and staff who had spent prior years providing "the Latino voice" in other organizations had the opportunity to take their experiences and expertise back to their otherwise neglected communities. As a coalition of groups completed a formal, state-sponsored study of Latino AIDS issues, one of the coalition's organizers told me, "After 15 years, the Latino community is going [to Albany] on its own."

"OTHER" NO MORE

The first wave of HIV/AIDS organizing had adopted a very broad focus, which gradually narrowed to a few key organizational forms and political postures—integrating with government services or opposing state policy—in the name of a few identified population categories. By the time people of color began forming their own HIV/AIDS organizations, the notion of AIDS work and the categories under which it was organized were becoming familiar to the state and the community. The reality had never been as clear cut as the labels would suggest, but people thought they understood the distinctions. Newer mobilizations, mostly occurring between 1985 and 1990, sought to provide representation and collective voice to everybody else. In doing so, the organizations struggled to explain to their constituencies, to their allies, and to potential funders who they were and why they needed to exist. They diversified the face of AIDS, expanded the definitions of response to the epidemic, and carved out new niches in the flow of people, ideas, and resources.

By 1985, most of the older service agencies, the empowerment groups, and almost all of the newer advocacy groups had formed women's groups within their own walls, but there were no women's organizations. Organizing for women affected by HIV/AIDS was difficult given the image of HIV disease. The fact that the official criteria for an AIDS diagnosis were based on the presentation of symptoms in men—thereby overlooking the most common early signs experienced by women—in addition to the routine exclusion of women from clinical trials, meant that many women with discernable HIV disease did not even know that women were susceptible (Berer 1993). Of greater concern, many of their doctors were equally ignorant. Up to that point, most of the women involved with the HIV/AIDS CBOs had joined as care providers for men. Through the various small groups within the larger groups, however, women began to develop their own picture of women's unique needs and risks.

As community organizations increasingly exchanged information on emerging patterns of infection, community-based efforts expanded accordingly. With the addition of women's organizations and Asian groups, the field began to define areas of work that had not yet been acknowledged at the federal level. Positioning themselves within the contours of the community-based organizational field, these new groups carved out spaces that no one else had defined, or wanted.

In the latter half of the 1980s, two women's groups began operating in New York City in separate niches. The primary missions of the Women and AIDS Resource Network (WARN, established 1986) were to distribute current and accurate information to affected women and to provide support for women facing HIV. Founded by Marie Marthe Saint Cyr, onetime director of the Haitian Coalition on AIDS, WARN began operating as an information clearinghouse on issues of HIV/AIDS in women's lives at a time when women in New York were just becoming the demographic group with the fastest-growing rates of new HIV infections.

Life Force—Women Fighting AIDS (1989) began as a demonstration project within a larger education association for health professionals. As the name implied, Life Force drew upon the advocacy and organization model of the empowerment movement. But their focus was on peer education, with women whose lives were directly affected by HIV reaching out to other women at risk or who were otherwise dealing with HIV/AIDS in their lives. Life Force was not particularly involved in either politics or service delivery. Their mission was to provide personal support through therapy and counseling, personal empowerment, and education.

The idea of "women fighting AIDS" was not a battle metaphor but a rallying call for women to work together against the misinformation that they,

their communities, and even their doctors possessed, and to counter the ideological "disinformation" that made it so hard for women to pursue HIV/AIDS
information. They assumed that much of the best information available from
other organizations was derived from, or centered on, the male experience,
and that it was therefore likely to overlook issues that women needed to
know. This information was not rejected but was filtered, annotated, and re-
worked to make it applicable to their target audience.

Between them, the two organizations began the process of reproducing on
a smaller scale the growth of an independent community space of work like
the one that had been built for HIV-positive men, while providing necessary
information about women and HIV to those other groups.

The empowerment movement that had worked to build communities of
support among people living with HIV/AIDS had, for the most part, been
speaking to the needs of young White men who lived alone, apart from their
families. With the greater awareness and involvement of women living with
HIV in the field, community organizers began to examine HIV/AIDS as a
family issue. Couples became infected together, leading to the prospect of
two sick or dying parents who, far from getting the help they needed, were
still striving to take care of their own children. Alianza Dominicana, in Washington Heights, began operating the first family care center in New York in
1987. The specific mission of the organization was to address unmet health
care and social service needs for Latino families, although they also undertook a great deal of prevention education. Yet Alianza did not officially begin
an HIV/AIDS program until 1989 with the receipt of their first AIDS Services
grant, choosing instead to define themselves as a family-based multiservice
center. Alianza positioned itself between local families, to whom they offered
outreach and education, and local hospitals, with whom they had formal linkage agreements. Unlike some of the larger organizations that were being
overrun with requests for services, Alianza was still recruiting clients into the
early 1990s. A project manager stated that funding was not too much of a
problem; ignorance about HIV was. "Families don't talk about it," he stated.
"People are very misinformed."

Further expansions of HIV/AIDS organizing would depend on contact with
existing networks of activists in other fields. The Asia Pacific Islander Coalition on HIV and AIDS aggressively sought to bring HIV/AIDS education and
prevention into their communities and their communities into the mainstream
health care system. Founded in 1989 as a pan-Asian umbrella organization,
they created a central point for HIV/AIDS services, education, advocacy, and
support. The original planners included members of the AIDS Coalition to
Unleash Power (ACT UP), NMAC, and GMHC,[1] as well as the city's Department of Health.

APICHA followed the pattern of the Latino organizations and the women's groups, defining its own culturally specific outreach efforts while aggressively representing its constituency in the HIV/AIDS policy and health care domains. A particular target of their lobbying was the Department of Health and Human Services' designation of Asian and Pacific Islanders as "other." The group's efforts were successful, giving them the responsibility to collect and propagate more data useful to both the state and their communities. A 1998 fundraising event, called "Other No More," celebrated the boundary-spanning activities of the group, which, according to APICHA's ten-year history, "helped to lessen the terrible isolation that Asians and Pacific Islanders confronting HIV and AIDS . . . experience."

Follow the Money

The rapid expansion of HIV/AIDS work into new niches both fostered and followed changes in the public response to AIDS. Specifically, most of the third-wave groups relied much more heavily on outside grants and government support than the earlier organizations had. They tapped into the growing public willingness to support community-based HIV/AIDS services and organizing that had been fostered by first- and second-wave groups. At the same time, they all faced the problem that the widespread understandings of what HIV/AIDS was and who it affected did not include any of them. They had to prove to both those outside the field and those within it that they were needed.

For many of the emerging organizations representing the "rest of the AIDS community," the measure of their success was their ability to work with health officials. Unlike the first groups, the organizations of the late 1980s defined their roles in the context of an existing space of work, one that had already garnered tens of millions of dollars in public and private funding. Also in contrast to the founding organizations, these later groups represented populations that tended to be resource poor. (This is not to endorse the stereotype, occasionally heard then, that all of the gay men in New York were rich. It's simply that some of them were, and many were both active and generous without much regard for class divisions.)

Cultural conflict notwithstanding, money has a great deal to do with who is or who is not able to organize an independent voice or mobilize large numbers of people in response to a social crisis. As noted in chapter 2, the mobilization of economic resources in communities of color followed the inroads into health and social service agencies that were pioneered by gay organizers and activists. Lacking a surplus of "indigenous funding," the minority groups were more dependent on state sources. Yet these same communities were more wary of co-optation. Existing public services had already failed to provide the kinds of support needed by an underserved, underinsured population. The organized community needed to do its own advocacy and activism work. Not surprisingly, however, the state's AIDS Institute had only committed to funding "local" service groups working in the "GMHC model." This organizational form was very client oriented and minimally political. A small wave of important community-based activity drew upon this funding, improving the health and knowledge of minority communities without greatly altering their clout. As the minority CBOs found footing in the domain of HIV/AIDS services, they remained second-class citizens on the political front.

The organizations of people of color all faced difficulty generating any community mobilization as long as HIV/AIDS could still be considered a gay problem. Yet the city funding on which they relied was for outreach and education, not research or advocacy, thereby limiting their ability to document community needs or define a larger minority agenda. Each limitation reinforced the other. "While a small number of African-American and Latino gay men were beginning to organize," Melinda Cuthbert noted, "they did so within the non-Latino White gay community. They joined existing groups at the Gay and Lesbian Community Center or volunteered at gay CBOs and continued to have very low visibility in their community" (1990, 205).

Despite the contradictions between activism and professionalism and between successful White advocacy and the relative invisibility of people-of-color communities, the professional image of the mainstream AIDS service organizations also encouraged the growth of new CBOs. "Once funding streams were in place, organizations serving people of color and injecting drug users turned to government agencies and to foundations because these sources were more accessible than individual donors" (Chambré 1997, 480). In other causes or other diseases, mainstream groups would often worry about being discredited by association when the poor, the homeless, and different ethnic groups sought to work with them. In this case, the more marginal segments of the field were able to take advantage of the mainstream image cultivated by the established groups, gaining access to the state or city departments of health by associating with established community organizations. And despite the ongoing criticism of its ethnic imbalances and dominance in the funding domains, groups like GMHC could still reasonably claim credit for increasing the pool of resources available to "the community" overall. "We've tried to seed other voices," one GMHC staff member explained. For example, MTFA, along with ADAPT, Momentum, PWAC/ NY, and other organizations with minority constituencies formed a temporary coalition with GMHC to lobby for more funding from the city and state (Chambré n.d., 31). This effort brought more money into the community, but only for GMHC-certified programs. Such collaborations also allowed GMHC to develop minority-directed programs of its own, and to legitimately apply for grants to run them. They increased their stature, reach, and resource base by sponsoring new groups and new initiatives.

The service community's greater reliance on public funds meant that groups had to constantly demonstrate that they performed unique and necessary services. The combined effect of this narrowing of catchment areas and the particularizing of organizational missions fostered a reshuffling of the field of CBOs as the decade drew to a close. The growth of women's advocacy efforts from existing service organizations provides a case in point. The AIDS Service Center (ASC) of Lower Manhattan split off from the Lower Manhattan AIDS Task Force in 1990 to provide a broader range of services within a more concentrated area. The HIV Law Project split from ASC in 1992, after which the Law Project helped to launch the Coalition for Women's Choice in HIV Testing and Care in 1996. ASC was primarily a service organization, which billed the city or the state for reimbursement for some of its services.

The HIV Law Project had begun informally as an advocacy project within the Mobilization for Youth Legal Services but not as its own organization and with no organizational "home." Having applied for AIDS Institute funding, they were told informally that they could receive support but only under the auspices of an already-funded CBO. The Law Project enrolled the support of ASC, which would provide a form of organizational endorsement. After some mission conflict, however, including lawsuits by the Law Project against some of ASC's funders, the Law Project returned to its original plan to work independently. As an interim measure, however, since the group needed a legitimate HIV/AIDS nonprofit to channel its funding, the Law Project grafted itself onto the Women's Prison Project. Once incorporated, the Law Project "split" from the Prison Project. The Coalition for Women's Choice, on the other hand, grew out of a response by the HIV Law Project to New York State's proposals for the mandatory HIV testing of pregnant women and newborns. This advocacy effort was organized as an independent coalition almost from the start in order to encourage greater participation without a predefined power structure. It therefore had to separate itself from the Law Project as quickly as possible. Although the Coalition of Women's Choice was a new entity, run by members of at least six other organizations, its genesis relied on the fluid movement of people, money, expertise, and other resources from group to group within the community network. Having emerged from an advocacy group working within a service group, the Coalition for Women's Choice drew significant support from the subfields of women's organizations, minority organizations, and activists.

SEEDING OTHER VOICES, 1987–1990

After some years of experience with community mobilization, members of the organized community began to concentrate on mobilizing other resources. That is, a number of private nonprofit organizations began to emerge whose primary mission was to help other groups. Industry-related HIV/AIDS groups, such as DIFFA (the Design Industry Foundation for AIDS), the Actor's Fund, Broadway Cares, and Equity Fights AIDS, took on responsibility for raising private funds within heavily affected arts-related professions. Whereas Broadway Cares (established 1986) hosted large fundraisers and provided grants of a few thousand dollars to local HIV/AIDS service organizations, Equity Fights AIDS (established 1985) collected smaller amounts and offered assistance to members of the profession who were living with HIV/AIDS. The two groups merged in 1987, since which time they have distributed hundreds of thousands of dollars through service organizations including AIDS Resource Center/Bailey House, Housing Works, God's Love We Deliver, and the Brooklyn AIDS Task Force.

Far more commonly, established groups supported the growth of the HIV/AIDS community by providing an organizational base from which new efforts could emerge. Housing Works, for example, grew out of the ACT UP working group on homelessness. Housing Works's executive director Charles King explained that the working group had found that a great many of the people with AIDS that they sought to represent were homeless and were thus facing discrimination on at least two fronts simultaneously. The fact that most of them were African American or Latino formed a "triple burden" in the social service world. Although there are many advocacy and help groups for homeless people in New York, none of them addressed the specific needs of people with HIV/AIDS. Furthermore, many of them refused to take on people with AIDS (PWAs) as clients (depending on the situations of their shelters and other resources, or just as a matter of discrimination). The group thus "discovered" a new arena of need within the AIDS community.

The core activists of the working group staged rallies and protest actions against the city's Division of AIDS Services (DAS) and the federal office of Housing and Urban Development (HUD). But many of the group's members, particularly those housing advocates whom ACT UP had recruited for the working group, sought to provide more tangible services. For this, they relied on grants and collaborations with the city and the state, including both DAS and HUD. A great many of the housing advocates were people of color who had come to this work as part of the larger project of collective action in impoverished minority communities.

While still a part of ACT UP, Housing Works had been almost entirely dedicated to activism. But their sense of mission shifted considerably once they began participating in national events on poverty and the homeless. In 1990, when the group chose to spin off an independent organization to provide housing for people living with HIV/AIDS, they took a step away from political disputes and AIDS activism into the domain of service provision. In practice, they also brought many former clients into the agency as volunteers, trainees, and staff. They located their work in the domain of housing, poverty, and racial discrimination, with a unique focus on HIV/AIDS rather than the other way around. Housing Works was thus born of an activist identity and actively sought to maintain its radical organizational identity while relying almost entirely on public support for a wide range of public service provision.

Like Housing Works, the People with AIDS Coalition of New York reorganized itself around issues that were of higher priority within communities of color. Both organizations committed themselves to a majority "minority" presence on their boards of directors. For PWAC/NY, this included publications written in Spanish, not translated from English for a Spanish audience; outreach into Harlem from their downtown offices; and research, support, and publications concerning prison issues. Like many of the groups located further from the center of the network, PWAC/NY defined itself in contrast to the core network functions. "PWAC is cool," a staff member explained. "We deal with issues that no one else will touch."

Both of these organizations sought to bring communities of color into the city's AIDS services system. Having defined populations of need and documented the specific needs of their populations, the minority-directed service organizations were able to compete for city contracts to address these needs. This first step defined communities of color as legitimate clients of the Department of Health. As community-based advocacy organizations, however, these same groups also defined their communities as contractors and as experts. Starting from a location outside of the system, at times opposing the city's policies and programs, they aggressively pursued insider politics.

Once the city had implemented programs for communities of color and a contracting mechanism to fund it, these sectors of the field grew more rapidly. New groups responded to calls for proposals and other externally driven opportunities that were specifically intended to generate work in new arenas. Iris House, a free, multiservice center for HIV-positive women and their families, was founded in 1991 with funding from the Manhattan Borough President's Office. Several of the task force CBOs (AIDS Center of Queens County, Staten Island AIDS Task Force, Upper Manhattan Task Force on AIDS, and the Bronx AIDS Services) were founded by social service professionals and funded by New York State to bring a community-based service model to communities that didn't already have one (Chambré 1997, 474). (Another interpretation is that in some of these communities, particularly with respect to services for drug users, the state was hesitant to recognize or fund the groups already doing the work and so created their own; cf. Perrow and Guillén 1990, 121.)

Gay Men of African Descent (GMAD) was created in 1986 in response to an AIDS Institute request for proposal (RFP). They attempted, with mixed success, to bridge the gaps among several identity statuses. For several years, the organization used city funds to do HIV/AIDS prevention education and outreach to African-American adolescents. Later, while the organization maintained a series of support groups and other meetings for men of all ages, an informant described the organization as "primarily a referral site." GMAD took in young gay men with concerns about HIV/AIDS and redirected them to more visible agencies but did not partner with those agencies in the definition or delivery of necessary services. Over time, the organization developed a host of in-house services and support groups and broadened its focus to all gay, lesbian, bisexual, and transgender (GLBT) people of color.

The fact that GMAD had no significant dealings with the largest "White" organizations likely further marginalized the group, as was suggested by respondents from other people-of-color organizations. GMAD existed in part because of the difficulties that African Americans living with HIV had in finding support and assistance from either traditional networks in their communities or existing AIDS service organizations. The CBO was created because its function was already somewhat marginal to the organized community. Unlike activist organizations for people of color, such as Harlem United and the National Minority Action Council, GMAD rarely participated in public activities relating to the collective identity of the network overall and was rarely referred to as a collaborator or resource by informants from other organizations.

The Brooklyn AIDS Task Force (BATF) also began as a response to a New York State AIDS Institute request for proposals in 1986, and the group functioned primarily as a service coordinator over a handful of semiautonomous programs. Most of their service programs were tied to local and federal funding. Yet the organization defined itself as a grassroots group creating innovative programs based on a culturally specific awareness of unmet needs. Throughout the 1990s, they used combinations of public and private funding to create new forms of support, outreach, and education to women, teens, and drug users.

Improved city funding created pockets of quasi-community-based organizations—nonprofit organizations situated in communities of need, with independent leadership structures, but almost totally dependent on public support. Although these groups were service oriented with little political involvement, they often remained highly embedded in their communities of origin and tightly bound to the community network. One BATF informant came to the organization as a development educator, paid by GMHC, to help BATF grow. In a little under a year, she left GMHC for a staff position at BATF. Her job represented a successful case of sponsorship of a new CBO by an established one, while both of the community groups are also fairly dependent on government support. BATF's location is defined somewhere between service and political advocacy, but their interorganizational relations are mostly formal, defined by the specifications of federal Ryan White CARE Act funding. BATF now has its own state-backed development program so that some external support still trickles down from them to newer organizations.

The Harlem United Community AIDS Center began as the Upper Room AIDS Ministry. Harlem United still provided pastoral care, but in their new form, they defined themselves as a multiservice center. Most of their work was coordinated through the local HIV Care Networks, service consortia funded at the federal level by the Ryan White CARE Act. They also worked with the city's Prevention Planning Groups. Informants report that funding changes increasingly forced service organizations to demonstrate that they could work together in a consortium structure, "to prove linkages." Through membership overlaps that are unrelated to the service consortia, Harlem United also undertook outreach to gay and transgender organizations in their community, increasing awareness of HIV/AIDS education, care, and services.

Organizations like Harlem United, which represented communities of color, experienced a number of awkward dependencies on other HIV/AIDS CBOs. As small "special interest" groups, they were unlikely to receive public support on their own, which pressured them into the service consortia. At the same time, many of their participants came to HIV/AIDS involvement through drug use, which meant that they often had criminal records and often were on parole or probation. This limited their potential activism. And, as representatives of resource-poor communities, they could not expect to raise enough money only within their own areas to support a fully independent mission. The combined carrot and stick of limited funding and criminal control of drug offenders required Harlem United, and others like them, to define themselves in relation to what others in the HIV/AIDS field were doing rather than breaking new ground. Yet many of these groups were created because of the sense that the existing groups did not want to do what the new organizers felt was most necessary.

What Was the Third Wave?

The emergence of smaller, more specialized organizations in the mid-1980s recognized and relied upon the institutionalization of community-based HIV/AIDS work within the state sector. As the most prominent and most recognized groups in the HIV/AIDS field had been moving toward a strategy of "normalizing" AIDS, these newer groups from different segments of the population were just starting to identify the needs of their communities and mobilize awareness. These third-wave groups followed the path already defined by the first two waves, but with two crucial differences. First, they were literally following a known path, not innovating and improvising. And second, they could draw upon both the accomplishments and the resources of the existing field.

The emerging organizations of and about women and people of color did not have to explain what HIV/AIDS was or say too much about how it was transmitted. They primarily had to convince their communities that everyone was at risk, that risk could be reduced, and that help was available for people who needed it. Their secondary positions in the HIV/AIDS field created a number of contradictions as they defined and expanded their missions and collective identities. By the time these groups began operating, the city and the state had created HIV/AIDS divisions and agencies, so they did not have to demand recognition from the public health sector. Yet these agencies had established connections with the existing community groups, including systems of financial support. The newer groups were less "competitive" in grant applications, having smaller constituencies and fewer accomplishments. Having entered the field later also hampered them.

With little regular access to support from the public health sector, the third-wave groups relied heavily on the support networks of the community-based field. Having these connections was necessary for their growth and survival. But it also fostered dependencies on their more established partners, creating conflicts over the different groups' influence in the overall community agenda. Experienced organizers who had worked with the larger groups were able to translate their expertise and connections into start-up efforts in the "other" communities. They launched their new groups with an already-defined place in the field and a preexisting set of interorganizational linkages. But by the same token, their strengths and their sense of mission were externally defined. The first-wave groups had built their organizations from the ground up, with only the help of their own communities. The later groups were working with multiple frames of reference and often had to "translate" outside information into a local context.

Having fewer people to draw upon, less money, and a less palpable sense of crisis, the emerging groups of this period could not realistically set out to do everything for themselves, nor did they need to. Their awareness of these conditions meant that less of their energy went toward justifying their existence and more into the traditional needs of developing and supporting an organizational infrastructure. They needed, and sought, outside funding.

Prior to the AIDS Institute requests for proposals, emerging groups had to rely on the sponsorship of existing community-based organizations in the HIV/AIDS field. GMHC's legal services department, which provides a variety of advocacy functions for PWAs and on behalf of all people living with HIV, was a particularly portable resource. Contacts associated with the Haitian Coalition on AIDS, Minority Task Force on AIDS, Bronx AIDS Services, and AIDS Center of Queens County (ACQC) have all acknowledged the regular support of GMHC's legal services for a variety of needs. The advent of state sources of funding allowed groups like GMHC to define services like those as community resources, available as needed, without having to take responsibility for the economic or organizational viability of the agencies they were assisting. That is, GMHC could get funding to provide "technical support" to other groups without either billing those groups or paying their startup costs. At the same time, the public health sector agencies that provided these grants could leave it to established AIDS service organizations (ASOs) to decide where and how this support could best be used. A large mechanism of public and private support grew up alongside the third-wave groups, and these groups could only choose whether or not to participate in it.

CBOs emerging from newly mobilized populations also looked for support from pre-HIV community groups involved with their constituencies. For the most part, such contacts produced no tangible results. The Minority Task Force on AIDS found that traditional funding sources were "hesitant to provide help when they were already funding GMHC." Consistently, these new CBOs fared better by establishing connections with the existing organizational base of HIV/AIDS organizations. Perceiving these established groups as "gay" rather than as AIDS specific, the people-of-color communities, injecting-drug-use supporters, alternative therapy groups, and women's organizations described their network-building activities as having to look outside of their communities for support but also as fighting to get their issues onto the agendas of the gay White men's groups. Both of these observations are accurate. By reaching into the network and *enrolling* HIV/AIDS CBOs for different kinds of work, the third wave of HIV/AIDS CBOs greatly expanded the scope of the network, diverting its course and reshaping its mission.

The third-wave organizations, therefore, initiated a reconfiguration of the network of community groups in a manner that forcefully altered relations between the state and community sectors. They entered a rather dense network of groups with a shared history that had cautiously staked out a limited set of relations with the public sector. These earlier groups represented "the AIDS community" to the state. They protected their autonomy as well as they could while still seeking support and occasional partnership opportunities from specific government agencies. Working through informal contacts and unofficial channels, the first- and second-wave groups that constituted the network had found ways to make themselves useful to public agencies without being answerable to them.

The third-wave groups expanded this work while throwing many of the working interorganizational relations into disarray. The newer groups treated both the community network and the state agencies as institutional sources of support. They partnered with both and applied for assistance from both. To the extent that the state and the community had come to accept a mainstream, normative definition of "the AIDS community," these newer groups challenged the working definitions of the field while serving and expanding upon its assumed purpose. That is, they did what everyone said needed to be done. They identified and sought out people in need, defined the unmet needs, and met them. Both the relevant state agencies and the established HIV/AIDS CBOs defined such work as fundamental to their missions. Yet the existence of these new groups as "outsiders" to an established field meant, uncomfortably, that the community and state groups had somehow become insiders together.

The ability of the third-wave groups to get public support meant that there was more support for the community. Their ability to define and reach different populations of need meant that the network was expanding and becoming more specialized. But it was the fact that these new groups worked with both state and community groups in similar ways that threatened to reduce the independence of the community network. The new groups were of the community and were tied to the state.

As noted, the existing organizations of the community network responded to these circumstances with some ambivalence. The larger groups defined outreach and "development" functions through which they were able to mediate between the state funders and the newer organizations. This partially addressed the concerns about independence and political autonomy as it gave the community groups more voice in defining which new needs were most valuable and which new organizations were most prepared to address them. This arrangement also suited the state agencies, such as the health departments and the AIDS Institute, since they were able to continue channeling most of their support through established and reliable service providers. In this way, the specialized division of labor within the network—represented by the new organizations and their "communities"—led to formal changes in the relations between the older private groups and the public health agencies. Necessarily, such hierarchical relations, made manifest in the flow of money from the state through the established network to the newer groups, revealed an increasing stratification of privilege within the community itself. It heralded a difficult, but crucial, period of growth for the organized community. The advent of this period of growth raised questions of coordination, control, and centralization that reverberated throughout the field.

Chapter 4 traces the complex organizational identity negotiations that followed from one such initiative as active drug users and their advocates sought to enter the field.

NOTE

1. ACT UP—the AIDS Coalition to Unleash Power—is discussed in chapter 7. GMHC, Gay Men's Health Crisis, and NMAC, the National Minority AIDS Council, are discussed in chapter 2 and earlier in this chapter.

Chapter Four

HIV/AIDS, Drug Use, and Zero Tolerance, 1985–1990

I was sitting at a street corner syringe exchange site in Harlem, one consisting of a van, two folding tables, and two staff members. I spoke with the male outreach worker in English. Local people occasionally approached the woman, conversed briefly in Spanish, and then counted out the used syringes they were dropping into the HazMat box in exchange for the same number of new ones. I mentioned to the man that they didn't seem to have a lot of visitors that day. "They keep asking if you're a cop," the woman responded. I skipped to my last few questions, exchanged business cards, and left. I thanked them for their time; they thanked me for leaving.

Throughout the HIV/AIDS epidemic, New York City has had the greatest number of cases of any city in the United States. Drug use surpassed other transmission routes as the leading source for new infections by 1992, and by the end of century was found to account for approximately 45 percent of known AIDS cases in the city (Bureau of HIV/AIDS Epidemiology 1999).[1] New York has consistently shown the highest rates of HIV infection among drug users compared with other U.S. cities. Yet HIV/AIDS prevention policies for drug-using populations have been limited at best.

The prevalence of HIV/AIDS among injecting drug users (IDUs) raised a number of difficult social, political, and public health questions. Within the public health sector, these questions occurred at the intersection of many much-older problems including disease prevention, poverty, racism, drug use, moral contests, long-term financial burdens, adaptation to crisis, and the inconsistent needs of public health versus law enforcement in policies concerning drug users. Underlying this conflict was the question of state support for private initiatives whose clients and participants are neither represented nor

83

desired in discussions of public policy. Proposals for controversial interventions such as syringe exchange—in which injecting drug users are given sterile syringes in exchange for used ones in order to reduce the transmission of HIV—generated tension between public health advocates and supporters of the war on drugs. Most significantly, efforts to implement syringe exchange forced us to confront our commitment to the welfare of a subpopulation defined principally by their association with a criminal activity.

Community-based nonprofit organizations working on behalf of injecting drug users had more hurdles to overcome than any single organizational effort could hope to meet. Organized primarily in low-income communities of color, their efforts were perceived as threatening to almost everyone involved and to many who weren't. Their success, to the extent that they succeeded, reflected a long period of creative accommodation, cautious self-effacement, and waiting for opportunities. Yet these opportunities did not merely arise through random interactions of social factors. Those organizations involved in syringe exchange and other HIV prevention work for drug users nurtured a set of relations and collaborations that created the opportunities they needed. This chapter explores the nature of this political environment and the community organizations' efforts to change it.

BARRIERS TO (HIV) PREVENTION

The association of HIV/AIDS with drug use posed a particular political threat to communities of color. Not wanting to search out homosexuality in their midst, political leaders of the African American and Latino communities in New York were slow to begin a conversation on HIV/AIDS. This absence left many watching with silent anxiety as professional commentators packaged AIDS, drugs, poverty, and race together in a familiar construct of the "self-destructive ghetto population." The proposal, by White leaders in the city and state departments of health, that syringe exchange programs could reduce "urban" HIV/AIDS rates was initially viewed as an insult, or worse. "[T]he majority of black elected officials and traditional black leaders, after evaluating the possible lifesaving benefits from a needle-exchange program to a largely black and Latino/a drug-using population and the minimal threat posed to nonusers in these same communities, sided with their black, nonusing, *voting*, and *morally upstanding* constituents" (Cohen 1999, 103, emphasis in original).

Black resistance to syringe exchange was not simply a matter of denial on the part of community leaders. These same leaders had long sought additional state and city resources for drug treatment in minority neighborhoods. The offer of free syringes for drug users, *instead of* the expansion of treatment services, easily fed into conspiracy theories and the very tangible distrust of government HIV policies among African Americans (Thomas and Quinn 1991). Anti-HIV mobilizing by and on behalf of people of color, straight or otherwise, was delayed by conflicting agendas, fear, and a lack of widespread attention to the issues.

Established organizations were also hesitant to take a strong position on syringe exchange, let alone to challenge existing drug laws. The closer the mainstream service agencies moved to legitimacy within the public health sector, the less they could afford to be tarnished by antigovernment protest actions and campaigns to organize drug users in New York City. In their place, current and former injecting drug users initiated HIV/AIDS outreach and prevention efforts on behalf of other users. These efforts coincided with the rise of AIDS street activism, and the user advocates found their allies there. Seizing the channels of elite access created by the service groups' limited partnerships with government agencies, activists and drug-user advocates initiated a pressure campaign to incorporate the least visible, least desirable citizens affected by HIV/AIDS into the country's slowly emerging prevention policies.

THE LATENT EFFECTS OF DRUG WARS

Injecting drug use was suspected as an HIV/AIDS transmission route early on in AIDS epidemiology. Although it had been listed as a risk category in 1983, drug treatment centers, home care agencies, and other health and service CBOs in New York City made no apparent accommodation to the discovery. In one of the few studies to examine organizational responses to HIV/AIDS in New York, Melinda Cuthbert (1990) found the drug treatment field unwilling to alter their normative state-funded practices in the direction of AIDS prevention or any other harm reduction work. State agencies adopted the same approach. "The New York State Division of Substance Abuse, . . . tiny and underfunded as it was, had many routes into the minority community; but like most organizations, it virtually ignored the problem for the first few years. Its mandate was to fight substance abuse, not the disease that was killing the abusers" (Perrow and Guillén 1990, 75).

Activists and advocates of HIV/AIDS prevention among drug users faced most of the same obstacles that the first wave of mostly gay community organizers had confronted. But with drug use, the problems were far more severe. Not only were the users themselves more hidden, more isolated, and with less social, political, and economic capital to mobilize, but the very structure of the law and social policy was becoming realigned into the largest "war" on drug use in the history of the nation. Whereas right-wing senators might have pushed the boundaries of casual discrimination by entering homophobic rhetoric into new legislation, there were no boundaries at all on hostility to drug users. From Jimmy Carter's failed reelection bid in 1980[2] and continuing unabated to this day, any politician who appeared "soft on drugs" became an easy target to a "tough on crime" opponent (Jensen and Gerber 1998, 19).

The conflation of behavior with identity has been more explicit in the case of injecting drug use than in any other part of the AIDS discourse and with a much longer history to draw upon. Drug users have long been "the other," representing a threat from a location that was necessarily separate from society. The public problem has never been *drug use* in America, which would imply that Americans used drugs, but *drug users*, who constituted a contagion, an alien agent weakening American society from within. In campaigns to alter public policy, antidrug activists have long emphasized the dangerousness, not of drugs, but of drug users (Lune 2002b). Injecting drug users in the early 1980s were not simply a marginal population; they were the enemy. No social ill, from increasing divorce rates to the crumbling urban infrastructure, was too obscure to be blamed primarily on drug use. Adding HIV/AIDS to the list merely confirmed the prevalent sense of drug users' culpability.

Antidrug rhetoric had begun in earnest during the debates surrounding the country's first national drug control law, the Harrison Act of 1914. Many of the terms and notions introduced nearly a century ago persisted through the decades of increasingly harsh and sweeping antidrug laws, and they remain in place today. Early twentieth-century campaigns against drug use focused on race almost exclusively, with interracial sexuality providing additional opprobrium. Opium supposedly lured "a large number" of White women into "living as common-law wives or cohabiting with Chinese," while "cocaine use [was] often the direct incentive for the crime of rape by the Negroes" (Gray 2000, 46, 47). During the red scare of the 1920s, drugs were described as a weapon by which foreign Communist subversives would undermine America's war readiness (Musto 1999). Congress was urged to action lest the addict become "organized and vocal," and "society might awaken to find that he is an IWW [Industrial Workers of the World], a bolshevik, or what not" (Musto 1999, 133).

Antimarijuana laws in the 1930s were fed by images of Mexican farm workers taking advantage of White women in the Southwest, not to mention taking White men's jobs. In 1937, Harry Anslinger, the head of the Federal Bureau of Narcotics from 1930 to 1962, wrote that under the influence of "the evil weed," marijuana, "much of the most irrational juvenile violence and killing that has written a new chapter of shame and tragedy is traceable directly to this hemp intoxication" (Anslinger and Oursler 1961, 38). Dramatic increases in the use of criminal sanctions and police violence against cocaine use in the 1950s followed sensational media stories of "cocainized Negroes" on rampages of raping and pillaging throughout the South.[3] In later years, similar fears of drug-addicted African Americans running through the streets looking for people to mug in support of their habits made urban ghettos a place of fear and repressive police control (Courtwright, Joseph, and Des Jarlais 1989). As Richard Nixon famously expressed it, "You have to face the fact that the whole problem is really the blacks. The key is to devise a system that recognizes this while appearing not to."[4] More recent changes in drug law and policy appear to have taken the Nixon mandate to heart. The crack hysteria of 1986, culminating in the introduction of the federal death penalty for "drug kingpins" and the longest mandatory minimum sentences ever for drug possession (for crack cocaine, but not powder cocaine), have been widely criticized as a war on African Americans (ACLU 1993; Duster 1997).

The antidrug discourse has always had a class-based component as well, which fed the conflict between medical and criminological approaches to drug control. Public health and criminal control strategies for drug addiction emerged together between 1910 and 1925. Each focused on the nature of addiction, and both approaches shared a basic taxonomy of types of addicts, summarized in a 1918 article in the *American Journal of Clinical Medicine*: "In Class one, we can include all of the physical, mental and moral defectives, the tramps, hoboes, idlers, loaders, irresponsibles, criminals, and denizens of the underworld. . . . These are the 'drug fiends.' In Class two, we have many types of good citizens . . . who are in every sense of the word 'victims' . . . doctors, lawyers, ministers, artists, actors, judges, congressmen, senators, priests, authors, women, girls, all of whom . . . want to be cured" (Duster 1970). Attention to the latter belonged to the public health sector, while the former, the majority, were the purview of its own branch of law enforcement. Thus, drug users were not criminals because they used illegal substances. It was well "understood" that most drug users were already criminal types, significantly involved in theft, murder, rape, socialism, and un-American activities. Drug use was presumed to be just another symptom of their illegitimate natures.

There have been attempts to criminalize drug addiction itself as an identity status, separate from drug use. Yet, due precisely to the legal distinction between behavior and identity, such laws have not endured. A State of California law criminalizing addiction was struck down in 1962 (Pascal 1988, 120), establishing a precedent on constitutional grounds. Much like homosexuality under antisodomy laws, the Supreme Court ruled that one can only be prosecuted for engaging in illegal acts, not for being the sort of person who would do that, or who has done so in the past. Similar attempts to criminalize homelessness throughout the country have been challenged or overturned for similar reasons (Ades 1989; Simon 1982).

Apart from the specific laws concerning the possession, sale, purchase, transportation, and consumption of controlled substances, most states and many cities have additional laws and ordinances restricting the possession of "drug paraphernalia" such as bongs, pipes, roach clips, syringes, cookers, and other implements that are designed to assist in drug use. In the United States, forty-nine states and Washington, D.C., have enacted drug paraphernalia laws, and many states have additional prescription laws concerning "dual use" items, notably syringes, which can have both legal and illegal purposes. On top of these restrictions, cities have created their own anti–head shop ordinances to shut down stores that sell uncontrolled drug-related items to people who might want to use drugs.

Despite the occasional constitutional challenge, these laws have proven quite resilient. After an initial series of paraphernalia laws were overturned, mostly for vague wording, the Drug Enforcement Administration developed the Model Anti-Paraphernalia Act to guide states in their efforts to implement regulations that will stand up in court (Tillett 1982, 2). Thirty-eight states and Washington, D.C., have based their laws on this act (Healey 1988, 1). (The Model Act itself was declared unconstitutional by the Sixth U.S. Court of Appeals in Cincinnati [Leonhardt 1980, 5], but with little long-term impact.) Paraphernalia laws and other restrictions on syringe possession rest on the premise that since there can be no legal justification for owning drug-related implements, their possession indicates the intent to commit a crime, which may therefore be treated as the initial stage in an unfolding criminal activity. Extending this logic slightly, drug users found carrying used syringes have been charged with drug possession based on the traces of drug measurable in the syringe (Abdul-Quader et al. 1999, 285). Such laws may be read as attempts to recriminalize addiction as an identity status, since they facilitate the prosecution of users who are not actually using drugs when arrested.

Under paraphernalia laws, it is not necessary to catch drug users in the act of purchasing, carrying, or using illegal drugs. If they are carrying drug paraphernalia, such as syringes, then they are subject to arrest. For drug users with previous arrests, this infraction is sufficient to revoke an existing parole or probation and could lead to lengthy periods of incarceration. It is paraphernalia control laws, not drug laws, that specifically mandate against syringe exchange programs.

THE CULTURAL POLITICS OF SYRINGE EXCHANGE

The strict criminal control perspective on drug policy in recent decades left little room for public health interventions. The White House Office of National Drug Control Policy (ONDCP), the federal government's primary anti-drug strategy office, has described syringe exchange and other harm reduction proposals as "a guise" under which secret plans to legalize narcotics will be set in motion (ONDCP 1999, 52). Conditions of parole and probation for convicted drug offenders have also kept many users out of treatment programs and away from community-based harm reduction facilities and syringe exchange programs. Since conditional release restrictions forbid drug offenders from associating with known users, they cannot enter community-based organizations that exist to serve them. "Drug-free zones" around schools also restrict the mobility of convicted drug offenders and therefore the placement of social service agencies.

The fear of arrest for syringe possession does not appear to have measurably reduced drug consumption, but it has discouraged injecting drug users from carrying clean needles (Bluthenthal et al. 1999). Instead, they had to either purchase syringes with the drug, which can be done in shooting galleries but rarely in the streets, or they reuse others' needles. "Syringes are shared because they are scarce, and they are scarce because they are illegal to possess without medical justification" (Koester 1994, 287). Since syringes are designed to capture, protect, and redistribute blood and bloodborne agents, syringe reuse has been a remarkably efficient means of HIV transmission.

In response to this situation, drug users and harm reduction advocates established syringe exchange programs (SEPs, or needle exchange programs, NEPs) in cities throughout the world. Injecting drug users can bring their used syringes to the exchange sites and swap them for sterile ones. The used equipment may be tested prior to safe disposal, by which means researchers track HIV prevalence among drug injectors. At most U.S. sites, users may also receive HIV tests if they wish or receive a referral for medical care or drug treatment, if available. But the primary benefit of SEPs is as an HIV/AIDS prevention measure. "As needles are removed from circulation (exchanged), the means of circulation time of the needles declines, which is associated with a decline in probability of infection. The provision of sterile needles in exchange for used ones reduces sharing, the number of times contaminated syringes are shared, limiting the number of viral transmission events" (Needle et al. 1998, 7).

The scientific element of the argument has not been the determining factor in syringe exchange policies (Moss 2000). For example, the U.S. Department of Health and Human Services Appropriation Act of 1998 indicated that federal support for syringe exchange would be withheld until the secretary determined that SEPs could reduce HIV without encouraging drug use. When the secretary of Health and Human Services made that determination later that year, the House of Representatives responded with a bill (HR 3717) to prohibit the use of federal funds in support of exchange programs regardless of the secretary's evaluation. Representative Newt Gingrich described the secretary's report as an endorsement of drug use that said "to every young person who is not sure, 'well, as long as your needle is clean, what's a little heroin or cocaine among friends?'"[5] Representative Mark Souder of Indiana created a moment of historical continuity by suggesting that needle exchange would enable heroin addicts to buy heroin, hit the streets, and therefore, commit rapes. "A woman gets raped in the street by a heroin addict. What are we going to tell her when she finds out that the needle . . . came from her tax dollars?" Notwithstanding Representative Nancy Pelosi's characterization of the debate as "a meeting of the Flat Earth Society," the measure passed overwhelmingly.

Syringe Exchange as a Community-Based Innovation

The world's first SEP was organized by Amsterdam's Interest Group for Drug Users (MDHG) in 1982.[6] With the recognition of HIV/AIDS as a public health threat to which injecting drug users were particularly vulnerable, the Amsterdam program gained municipal partnership by 1984, and the Dutch government adopted needle exchange as a formal nationwide policy in 1985 (Buning, Brussel, and van Santen 1992; MDHG 1992). Sweden and Australia followed suit in 1986, England and Scotland the following year. As in the Netherlands, the English and Swedish syringe exchange programs were initiated by users' groups prior to state involvement (Joseph and Des Jarlais 1989).

In many ways, the first SEP was the least controversial. Drug use in Amsterdam and drug-related health concerns were viewed primarily as problems belonging to the user community. To the extent that drug use was associated with crime, illness, or tourism, the police, the Municipal Health Services, and the city council would negotiate an appropriate response with the MDHG. "Drug tourists" from neighboring countries would often be picked up by the police and handed over to private service agencies, which would send them home. As long as the Municipal Health Services validated the MDHG's interventions, the police were content to let the community keep things under control.

SEPs in New York did not fare quite so well. SEP policy debates in New York were contentious from the start, with AIDS activists opposing elected officials, and public health officials divided or mute. (Several of the New York political and community leaders who initially opposed syringe exchange, including Congressman Charles Rangel and Reverend Al Sharpton, have since reversed their positions. Others are reputed, by informants for this study, to have changed their positions privately, but not for attribution.) When the Department of Health proposed implementing a pilot syringe exchange program in 1985, there was no attempt to involve IDUs or their advocates in its planning or implementation. This proposal was opposed by the police, the district attorneys of all five boroughs, many community leaders, most community boards in the directly affected neighborhoods, the local media, and the Catholic Church, among others. "Law enforcement officials immediately called the experiment 'unthinkable,' and many of the city's minority leaders denounced it as genocide" (W. Anderson 1991, 1506).

The Health Department plan called for five exchange locations throughout the city, each within a high HIV-seroprevalence area with known drug-using populations, but each also targeting a different community with slightly different combinations of services and outreach. Responding to popular concerns that SEPs would draw drug users into target neighborhoods, the mayor sought to reduce the number of sites supported by the program. Among other restrictions, the city mandated that no SEP could open within walking distance of a public school. Ultimately, due to these restrictions, only one site was opened, at the Department of Health headquarters across the street from One Police Plaza (referred to by one critic [McDermott 1992] as "the highest concentration of narcotics detectives in the western world"). Potential participants were accepted only by referral from the waiting lists of drug treatment programs, in part to ensure that participants would not include new users lured into drug use by the promise of free syringes. Those accepted had to carry photo ID cards identifying them as injecting drug users and submit to medical exams that included blood testing. Returned syringes were tagged and tested, and participants faced sanctions if blood-type testing indicated that they had allowed others to use their syringes.

A cordon of police stood by on the program's opening day, anticipating crowds of users and their antagonists, but the event was strangely quiet. Eight users applied to enter the program within the first week. "After two months . . . only 76 needles had been dispensed" (W. Anderson 1991, 1512). A year later, with the election of David Dinkins as the city's new mayor and the subsequent appointment of a city health commissioner "ideologically opposed" to syringe exchange (W. Anderson 1991, 1514), the program was terminated.

Community-Based Syringe Exchange Comes to New York City

In 1985, as HIV/AIDS prevention efforts in the gay community were beginning to show results, activist Yolanda Serrano began a collaboration with the sociologist Samuel Friedman to address the problem of HIV/AIDS among drug users. Friedman had studied the formation of drug-user interest groups in the Netherlands, and he advocated a model of self-organization and self-help for injecting drug users in New York. Serrano had been on the board of directors of ADAPT (the Association for Drug Abuse Prevention and Treatment), a community-based service group for drug users that had all but ceased functioning in the early 1980s. Serrano revitalized and reorganized ADAPT along lines influenced by the MDHG, the Dutch drug-user unions, but with adjustments for the more strict antidrug legal system in New York. Many elements of this plan did not succeed, but ADAPT became the first HIV/AIDS community-based organization (CBO) committed to harm reduction in New York (see Friedman and Serrano 1989).

ADAPT, a relatively small organization, pushed for drug law reform, particularly syringe exchange. Informants describe the work of the group as very hands-on, very personal with the injecting drug users for and with whom they worked and much less attached to the Department of Health (DOH). When ADAPT sought city funding for their HIV/AIDS prevention work, "the DOH refused because the organization was distributing bleach kits [for cleaning syringes] and thus 'encouraging' addiction" (Perrow and Guillén 1990, 120). An ADAPT organizer explained that, in his view, city officials wanted their work to fail. There was "no war on drugs. It's a war on people." ADAPT expected little help from the law or the city, and was prepared to oppose both.

Although the city Department of Health had proposed the New York City needle exchange trial program in 1985, by January 1988 the plan had yet to be approved by the state. ADAPT and the Hispanic AIDS Forum, among others, endorsed the proposal, but progress appeared to be stalled. According to outreach workers at ADAPT, Serrano then announced that in order to bring attention to the issue she would personally go into shooting galleries and hand out syringes until the city took action. Mayor Ed Koch publicly promised that Serrano would be arrested on the spot if she tried it, but he and city health commissioner Stephen Joseph used the occasion to criticize the governor and the state health commissioner for blocking the city's needle exchange trial (Joseph 1992, 199). Three weeks later, the state approved the syringe exchange plan. Whether the timing was coincidental or the state simply did not wish to allow a test case at that time, ADAPT's activism provided support for the unpopular health measure. The city's needle trial would ultimately be declared a failure, but supporters of community-based activism for syringe exchange claimed their first victory just for getting it opened.

Politics and Health Advocacy

Each of the SEPs currently operating in New York City under the state's waiver began as an illegal, underground exchange. They owe their existence to the intersection of three channels of organizational activity. One was the

AIDS Coalition to Unleash Power New York's (ACT UP/NY's) commitment to political activism. Another was ADAPT's AIDS prevention and harm reduction work, which an ADAPT worker claimed had "opened the door for ACT UP to do underground distribution." In between the two was the arrival of Jon Parker in New York. Parker, a needle exchange activist from New Haven who had been arrested multiple times in several states and was a founder of the National AIDS Brigade (NAB), began distributing syringes in Brooklyn, as much an act of protest as a health measure. ACT UP/NY quickly recruited Parker and Rod Sorge, a former heroin user, to help shape a new working group on needle exchange.

Parker and Sorge resembled the ACT UP constituency reasonably well. Both were White educated social outsiders with a commitment to political activism. Sorge was openly gay. But they were not typical of New York City's addict population. Invited by the needle exchange working group to address ACT UP's general meetings, organized drug users described the "uneasy interactions that took place" there. Many of them felt awkward and unwanted. An ACT UP member described an "uneasy alliance" after "the whole drug-using community" began to participate in ACT UP meetings.

An activist from ACT UP who had worked with the National AIDS Brigade recalled that there were "a lot of distractions" in the efforts of the group, through Parker, to collaborate with ACT UP. "NAB had a public health model. ACT UP had a political agenda." One of the implications of these differences was that while the NAB workers pushed the boundaries of the law and often sought to get the charges dropped when they were arrested, ACT UP was looking for a good show trial through which to challenge the laws.

ACT UP began supporting or operating irregular needle exchange efforts as a political act. They joined Parker in Brooklyn, where they would later be joined by ADAPT. Sorge worked with others who were trying to establish NEPs in Manhattan and helped to start new projects in the Bronx that would eventually seed the St. Ann's Corner of Harm Reduction (SACHR) and the Bronx-Harlem Needle Exchange, now called New York Harm Reduction Educators (NYHRE). The activists were committed outsiders, confident that they were helping, yet occasionally seen as colonial in their demeanor. "The fact that it was illegal to provide sterile injection equipment to drug users enhanced the credibility of the exchanges and served as a strong bond between the participants and the staff," researchers noted (Henman et al. 1998, 399).

But the ACT UP working group had more knowledge of legal challenges than of drug use. They didn't always ask or investigate where or how their efforts could best serve the communities on whose behalf they had mobilized. According to a SACHR staff member who had been with the original activists, "We ha[d] a bunch of people that just stand around and hawk bleach kits [for cleaning syringes] and wait, and bemoan how *these people* are not coming to the table and how *different* they are." Volunteers handed out syringes to noninjecting users who would later sell them to the IDUs. The activists didn't care how the mechanism worked as long as it got the needles into circulation. "It was good that they were doing this, but . . . they were just being activists. They weren't trying to do a service."

The initial distribution efforts were limited and uncoordinated. "The ACT UP NEP relies on the 'grapevine' method to spread the word," Richard Elovich and Sorge wrote. "Most of the newcomers to the program are brought by people who already use it" (1991, 170). The activists gave news interviews and wanted to bring camera crews to the sites, but the drug-user advocates opposed any such visibility. Underground SEPs, which tended to operate through inconsistent walking routes and irregular hours, were limited by the desire to remain inconspicuous, even in areas where they were unofficially tolerated by police. Joyce Rivera, the founder of SACHR, explained, "Both exchanges had a 'Brigadoon' aspect, a discretely organized social service entity that appeared weekly in a public landscape."

The ACT UP needle exchange workers decided to increase the stakes, and in April 1990, they took out an ad announcing their intent to distribute clean needles for free on the Lower East Side. The announcement listed the time and place, guaranteeing press coverage and leading to the immediate arrest of ten volunteers. At their trial, the activists entered a "necessity defense," arguing that given the rate of HIV infection among injecting drug users, their actions were necessary to save lives.

ACT UP's confrontational tactics had, in a sense, been leading up to this event. Former health commissioner Stephen Joseph, a longtime target of activist ire, was called to testify on behalf of the activists. "In my testimony I stated that the closure of the city's official needle exchange program left the defendants no choice but to take the actions that they did" (Joseph 1992, 220). The court agreed, declaring them "not guilty by public health necessity."[7]

The exact impact of the trial is difficult to gauge, but the court decision provided additional justification for the state Department of Health to endorse syringe exchange. According to a syringe exchange staff member at ADAPT, the trial created the opportunity to press for changes in the law that ADAPT had already been pursuing. "As part of a 'health emergency' declared by the Commissioner of the State Department of Public Health, the 'underground' exchange programmes were permitted to obtain 'waivers' exempting them and their participants from the legal requirement for prescriptions in the dispensing of sterile injection equipment" (Henman et al. 1998, 398). Through the waiver system, the state effectively circumvented the city's paraphernalia laws by defining conditions under which the local law would not be applied.

The trial may have been an important event for the political viability of the waiver, but some informants feel that it "did nothing for needle exchange." Most of the details concerning state regulation of community-based exchange programs had already been negotiated between New York State and AmFAR, the American Foundation for AIDS Research. AmFAR provided the funding for the quasi-legal exchange programs, since Congress had forbidden the use of federal funds for syringe exchange. The Department of Health agreed to grant a waiver to any applicant for AmFAR funds that met the criteria specified in their program application, which they had helped to define. The trial and subsequent waiver system legally established that the organized community could continue their privately funded activities on behalf of public health with minimal support or interference from the state. Furthermore, since the waiver system was backed by the state Department of Health's declaration of a health emergency, local police, prosecutors, and the mayor could all protect themselves politically by depicting syringe exchange as having been imposed on the city against their will.[8]

DIVISION OF LABOR AND
THE GROWTH OF SYRINGE EXCHANGE

The legal and extralegal battle over HIV/AIDS prevention policies for injecting drug users reveals a crucial element of the interorganizational relations within the organized AIDS community and between them and the state. Prior to HIV/AIDS, a broad spectrum of private drug-related agencies had grown in the city, supported by local, state, and federal government spending. With the advent of HIV/AIDS, none of these organizations would take a leading role in doing what the state chose not to do. New CBOs, organized around HIV/AIDS and with ties to the AIDS service organizations and the people with AIDS (PWA) empowerment movement, set out to define a new policy agenda for prevention and protection among drug users. These new groups introduced harm reduction concepts to the discussion and took steps to implement them. Yet, dependent on their tax-exempt statuses and with obligations to their clients, none of these advocacy-oriented service providers could afford to disobey the law or especially to get caught. Instead, they relied on the independent, confrontational ACT UP to press the issues. In the meantime, and behind the scenes, the drug-related HIV/AIDS CBOs provided support to the ACT UP syringe exchange underground.

The activist groups had no clients, no legal privileges, and no external dependencies. They were also peopled with young, angry, and mostly HIV-positive supporters. Many of these activists were wholeheartedly committed to HIV/AIDS politics, and for those who were falling ill, they often felt that they had little to lose through their actions. They repeatedly placed their personal freedoms on the line in order to challenge policy, to draw out supporters from the public health sector, and to test the extent of police and prosecutors' opposition. A great many of the political opportunities that service and advocacy groups found in the late 1980s were created by the high-risk activism of ACT UP/NY and their supporters. Their mostly nonviolent civil disobedience and colorful publicity stunts pressured the state at numerous points, altering the configuration of state-community relations.

The years following the introduction of the waiver system in 1992 were described by an activist as a "transitional moment for ACT UP." Some volunteers and exchange workers left the group to do full-time syringe exchange with the new programs that ACT UP had been supporting. The ACT UP/NY syringe exchange working group expanded into "two communities of color" on the lower east side and in the Bronx, making "alliances with people who didn't have an affinity with ACT UP." One formerly underground group joined with the Lower East Side Services Center to form the Lower East Side Needle Exchange Program. In the Bronx, Rod Sorge led the reorganization of an illegal program into the Bronx-Harlem Needle Exchange, later reorganized as the New York Harm Reduction Educators. Brian Weil transformed another underground exchange into CitiWide Harm Reduction. Joyce Rivera, a public health researcher who had been working with the activists, founded St. Ann's Corner of Harm Reduction. Each of them siphoned off some of the activists from ACT UP while recruiting interested active and former IDUs to staff their new CBOs.

Two additional CBOs, Positive Health Project (PHP) and ADAPT, operated syringe exchanges in Manhattan. Neither of these agencies was technically a spin-off from ACT UP, although they were connected to the activist community. PHP was founded in 1993 by Jason Farrell, a former IDU who had learned of syringe exchange at an ACT UP meeting in 1990. Farrell had worked as an underground exchange volunteer until he left to form his own service-oriented agency. ADAPT, having served as a syringe exchange catalyst early on, had no formal relationship with ACT UP or its underground exchange sites, though individual volunteers were active in both groups. ADAPT began operating its own SEPs in 1992.

An outreach worker at Harlem United credited ACT UP's work on needle exchange but stressed that the group lacked cultural sensitivity. "They don't hear the Black perspective on drugs in the community." A former ACT UP activist whom I encountered working at a buyers' club, had also voiced this criticism. "You shouldn't be in the Bronx unless you're willing to stay in the Bronx and do work." At the same time, when Harlem United and several other CBOs joined ACT UP for their "Target City Hall" event, it was the ACT UP contingent that moved forward to be arrested when confronted by the police. Harlem United could only participate in the protest action, volunteers explained, because other activists were willing to face criminal charges on their behalf.

The waiver system allowed and encouraged organizations conducting underground syringe exchange to come in from the cold. With the fewer legal restrictions, program organizers and participants were relatively free from the threat of arrest, though imperfectly so (Case, Meehan, and Jones 1998). But the waiver also meant that their very purpose was still illegal. They could not advertise, openly recruit participants, or press for greater support from the city (Lune 2002a). The ambiguous legal status of SEPs limited their growth; it served to "deter government health agencies and private parties from conducting syringe exchange, . . . deter government agencies and foundations from funding syringe exchange, and . . . prevent publicly funded syringe exchanges from getting liability insurance, charitable tax status, and other items necessary for effective operation" (Burris et al. 1996, 1161). The year following authorization of the first five programs, in 1992, only two additional waivers were granted. Two more waivers were issued the following year, and none since then. Several organizations continued to operate underground exchanges.

SURVIVING A HOSTILE CLIMATE

Even after the state waiver, SEPs were vulnerable to police, community, and media harassment. Informants reported witnessing police seizing or tearing up participants' ID cards while arresting them for syringe possession. Informants at ADAPT described how, following the opening of an exchange site in Brooklyn in the late 1990s, local police would follow the participants, waiting for them to purchase drugs. The exchange program "exposed participants to law enforcement," creating new problems and driving users back to the shooting galleries. Years later, long after the police changed their policies and generally seemed to support the program, street workers at ADAPT reported that only a small percentage of participants at the exchange were from the neighborhood.

Each of the groups still operating had successfully negotiated with the communities in which they worked and with local law enforcement. Relations were arranged with each precinct individually. Police often drove by to briefly observe the exchange operations, though rarely to harass anymore. Many of the beat cops knew the exchange workers and some of the IDUs by name and would stop to make sure the workers were not experiencing any trouble out on the streets, from either clients or local residents. Program staff encouraged the police to take HIV/AIDS education materials and condoms for their own use. Some traveled to the different precincts giving workshops on safe syringe disposal, or gave "sharps" disposal containers to police to carry in their cars. This form of exchange reduced the fears that police and IDUs had toward one another. Even so, there was always tension.

All of the programs stressed invisibility rather than outreach. In response to a question about neighborhood reactions to their mobile van, an informant at FROST'D (Foundation for Research on Sexually Transmitted Diseases) replied, "I don't think people know we're there." A source at another agency specified that they were a "multiservice" organization and would never hang a sign over their door that said "AIDS." When the programs expanded, they attempted to negotiate an invitation from their target community before moving in. Informants at two organizations discussed successful instances in which local elites arranged to have the syringe exchange program brought in with minimal contention. One program added a new street site within their catchment area at the request of the local police. And several informants at different organizations, each emphasizing that this was not for personal attribution, discussed the need to negotiate with local drug dealers for permission to operate on their turf.

In the early days of the Bronx-Harlem exchange, there was "no need for elite allies." The message to the Dinkins administration was "Just leave us alone." The goal of SEP interactions with the city was to "get Dinkins to not oppose it." When they needed additional funding for ancillary health services at the exchange sites, they "sought personal connections through informal networks." Even throughout the Giuliani administration, however, the Bronx-Harlem exchange program found "a lot of people in policy making positions" who "can't say so in many words but they can help you out." There are "people who are willing to meet with you in some restaurant in Morningside Heights" as long as they don't have to take a position publicly. Working through such contacts, SEPs tried to forestall each new threat as it developed. An informant from ADAPT stated that they communicated with politicians as part of their work. "They support us in private, but only tolerate us in public."

Significantly, given the political uncertainty surrounding their work, sources at many of the exchange programs complained about their inability to integrate their work into that of non-HIV–related organizations. SEPs define themselves as a bridge to treatment and other services, but other agencies involved with drug use keep their distance from the SEPs. Several informants indicated that they regularly referred clients to other service agencies but did not get referrals in return. The New York Academy of Medicine syringe exchange study anticipated this difficulty, noting that "some SEPs and abstinence-based drug treatment or social service providers see themselves as ideological contestants, rather than collaborators, in service provision to IDUs" (Finkelstein and Vogel 1999, 8). As one project director stated, "It's pretty much of a one-way relationship between syringe exchange and the larger service system."

Syringe exchange in New York was born of activism, but it is no longer an area of social movement activity. A few of the staff workers at different agencies, particularly those with a history of street activism for syringe exchange, were critical of the professional distance between the groups. But most of the newer leaders echoed the sentiment that they "have to become less ideological, or we condemn ourselves to the margin." In this, they have chosen to follow the path of the mainstream HIV/AIDS service organizations and to further "normalize" HIV within the public health sector.

Syringe exchange programs depend upon the ongoing support of city agents, including the police, the mayor's office, the city council, and local district representatives. While the programs have been endorsed by city, state, and federal health officials, almost no elected official has been willing to visibly support them while in office. Longtime participants, those who have made the transition from activism to services, see this as a defining condition for the operation of all SEPS. "There is no support from elected officials, or minimal. I can think of some city council members, and some state assembly people, and some state senate people, who've actually been outspoken in their support of the idea of syringe exchange. . . . So I won't say that it's completely hostile. But those guys are definitely operating in a hostile environment."

SEPs won the right to be tolerated but with the understanding that they could be shut down any time the state withdrew its unusual protection. SEPs were effectively excluded from much of public health services and the drug treatment field. Publicly supported health service agencies, including hospitals and drug treatment programs, could potentially be accused of violating the terms of their funding if they were to refer clients to a syringe exchange program. As a result, SEPs could not exist without public support from the institutional forces most clearly antithetical to them.

Despite the institutional incompatibility, syringe exchanges were able to collaborate with state agencies. SEPs and government agencies shared an interest in depoliticizing the programs. Many elected officials and most public health officials recognized the role of syringe exchange in limiting HIV transmission, just as program organizers recognize the political liability inherent in supporting them. The experience in New York City suggests that political opposition to SEPs derived more from the unpopularity of their constituency than from disagreement with the basic social role of SEPs. The problem was one of political accountability. Within both city and state government, SEPs found closeted supporters. As SEP advocates and organizers moved away from visible challenges in the political domain, government agencies responded by providing other points of access.

The Realpolitik of State-Community Relations

The circuitous path by which syringe exchange came into being demonstrates one of the key political functions of community-based organizations. The wave of activism that generated syringe exchange programs in New York required more involvement from state agencies than any previous expansion of the field. Yet most of the interactions between the community groups and their supporters at the state level concerned strategies for keeping the state out of the way. The privately organized, privately funded groups operating the SEPs allowed the state to offload responsibility for a necessary but politically hazardous public health service. Enough legislators and public health officials recognized the need for the service to create a hidden channel for support of the SEPs. As long as responsibility could not be traced back to anyone who needed to be elected, the government could allow it to happen.

For any existing organization, this arrangement has obvious merit. But the pragmatic, short-term benefits carry a considerable political cost. With a legislative sword of Damocles hanging permanently over their heads, exchange programs did what they could to ensure their survival, which necessarily entailed a depoliticization of their work. The integration of the former underground movement into the margins of the public health care system placed significant barriers between the advocates and their communities. What was once the syringe exchange movement in New York City distanced itself from the population in whose name they act. Having won the right to exist, they retreated from pursuing virtually any other (political) goal. Thus SEPs had to participate in their own marginality and invisibility as a condition for what amounts to a reduction of hostilities with state agencies.

Comparable politics and compromises colored the slow integration of SEPs into the HIV/AIDS community network. Drug users were even more socially and politically marginalized than the other mobilized groups. For activists, this made syringe exchange the perfect issue with which to demonstrate their commitment to public health while exposing the hypocrisy of the political world. For service providers with state contracts, this made syringe exchange the one issue that could by itself destroy their accomplishments. After ten years of careful work building popular sympathy for people with

HIV/AIDS, gay or straight, immigrant or native born, they were not quite prepared to link their fortunes to the public image of drug injectors.

Informants at the syringe exchange programs tended to be cautious about their claims, if not actually cynical or worse. They named "enemies" who worked against them. They spoke of their work as the thing they were able to do for the moment, as though it would all be crushed in the near future. Given all of the forces aligned against them, the success of syringe exchange advocates is hard to fathom. Yet they have been incredibly successful. Their first surprising accomplishment is that they exist. They have maintained their existence through years of difficulty and challenges from an ever-changing array of journalists, public officials, and community activists. Given the relative silence on the issue for the past several years, it appears that they have outlasted their critics. Syringe exchange has become fairly uncontroversial. This fact alone means that their public supporters can come out of the closet.

A second measure of their success is that syringe exchange programs have established a recognized niche within the community network. Resource guides published by the larger service organizations list exchange sites and contact information. The courtesy stigma that initially threatened the community has come to little, and so they too can openly endorse the principle of public health care and HIV/AIDS prevention for active drug users. Individual informants have moved from other segments of the field into syringe exchange work, and SEP activists have likewise integrated into new jobs elsewhere in the organized community.

Beyond the circumstances of their own organizational survival, however, SEP advocates have spearheaded legal changes that were unthinkable before the advent of syringe exchange. Their demonstration that access to needles had no visible negative consequences for the "war on drugs" became the basis for the new needle laws in New York State. In 2001, syringe possession was effectively decriminalized through the Expanded Syringe Access Program (ESAP), which allowed adults to purchase syringes over the counter in pharmacies.[9]

The existence of the ESAP means that (1) injecting drug users can get syringes without a prescription and that (2) needle laws are further superceded so possession has been decriminalized, from which it follows that (3) health officials can advise users to buy clean needles. In effect, the needle exchange movement has won, even though syringe exchange programs are still relatively invisible and syringes are still reused among IDUs. One can describe the changes that led to the adoption of ESAP in New York strictly in terms of public health and the responsiveness of political leaders to the recommendations of health leaders. Such a description would be misleading. Community-based SEP advocates, a new kind of public health activist, worked for years to create the conditions under which this could occur. They fought against nearly a century of hostile anti-drug-use legislation and a modern war on drugs campaign. They pressured medical professionals into taking a position on critical legal questions. They allied themselves with existing HIV/AIDS groups, using these groups' political connections to build a secret network of support within government and the health care system. They spent more than ten years creating the circumstances that allowed others to bring about the changes that they wanted.

Within the HIV/AIDS field, the initial attempts to integrate work on behalf of drug users with the larger set of community pursuits were awkward and isolated. ADAPT, for example, mostly worked on its own for years before ACT UP and AmFAR took up their cause. The main difficulty appears to do with state-community relations. SEP advocates took an oppositional stance to the state and were often seen and treated as criminals by state officials. This was not a position that the service groups and others that maintained working relations with government wanted to take. On the other hand, this was exactly the position that ACT UP wanted, even to the point where the activists became too oppositional for the drug users. Tempered and legitimated by their victory in court and by the new waiver system, SEP advocates finally achieved working connections with potential supporters throughout the HIV/AIDS world and with policy makers and health officials. With the state Department of Health openly supporting syringe exchange, it became safe for community service groups and drug treatment providers to do so as well. Finally, with Black and Latino groups taking over the exchange sites in Black and Latino neighborhoods, a dense, interconnected web of social actors aligned around the issue.

NOTES

1. The actual date at which HIV rates among IDUs surpassed other risk categories might have been much earlier. Rand Stoneburner et al. (1990) have argued that HIV rates among IDUs were dramatically undercounted throughout the 1980s.

2. Carter met with drug policy reformers and openly considered the decriminalization of marijuana.

3. "The fear of the cocainized black coincided with the peak of lynchings, legal segregation, and voting laws all designed to remove political and social power from [black men]. Fear of cocaine might have contributed to the dread that the black would rise above 'his place,' as well as reflecting the extent to which cocaine may have released defiance and retribution. . . . One of the most terrifying beliefs about cocaine was that it actually improved pistol marksmanship. Another myth, that cocaine made blacks almost unaffected by mere .32 caliber bullets, is said to have caused southern

police departments to switch to .38 caliber revolvers. These fantasies characterized white fear, not the reality of cocaine's effects, and gave one more reason for the repression of blacks" (Musto 1999, 7).

4. The text is an entry in H. R. Haldeman's diary, quoted in Jensen and Gerber 1998, 13.

5. Statements by representatives concerning HR 3717 were reported on *The News-Hour with Jim Lehrer*, April 29, 1998.

6. It is common to cite 1984, the year that the Dutch state first formally recognized syringe exchange, as the date of origin. However, IDUs in Amsterdam had already been operating a self-organized, self-supported program of distribution of sterile syringes, mostly stolen from the Municipal Health Services, as protection against hepatitis since late 1982 (author interview, MDHG, 1999). G. V. Stimson has indicated that injecting drug users had "some form" of syringe exchange available in the UK in the late 1960s. See Stimson et al. 1988.

7. *State of New York v. Bordowitz*, Criminal Court of City and County of New York, no. 90N028423 (June 25, 1991).

8. Eventually, in 1992, Mayor Dinkins reversed his opposition to syringe exchange, but quietly and with the visible encouragement of the city's new health commissioner and the Black Leadership Coalition on AIDS (Kirp and Bayer 1993, 89).

9. Expanded Syringe Access Demonstration Project, 10 NYCRR 80.137.

Chapter Five

The ACT UP Years

Following an ACT UP protest event in 1994, the group held a postmortem meeting. They discussed the reactions and fallout from their various targets, allies, and audiences, and they notably took the event organizers to task for exceeding their budget—that is, for not being better project managers. As one man stood in front of "the floor"—the scores of members in attendance that night—and walked them through his expense report line by line, he received the same angry treatment as some of their protest targets. "What about the taxi rides?" someone called out. There were so many things to transport, he explained defensively, uptown and back. Sounds of unrest. "Why not use the subway?" There wasn't time, he argued. "Besides, it's tiring, and I do have AIDS," he began, but the murmuring only grew louder. "Who doesn't?" someone shouted.

The first wave of community-based organizing had offered to work with the state and the public health sector but had been rebuffed. They would have worked as insiders had they been allowed inside. The second wave, the empowerment years, expanded the sense of community, mobilized a broader constituency, and concentrated on developing indigenous resources. These organizations were mostly independent of the state, staffed by people affected by HIV working for people affected by HIV. During the third wave, the organized community intensified its networking activities, connecting with other groups in both the private and public sectors, moving resources across cultural and organizational boundaries, and pressing the case that the government had an obligation to assist their private efforts as they fulfilled what were essentially public functions. These organizations were outsiders to the public health and policy domains but were relatively inward looking. Deeply embedded within their communities of origin, they defined the needs of their constituencies, and they defined their own responses to those needs.

The fourth wave, political activism, directed its resources against the state. The activists placed responsibility for the response to HIV/AIDS back in the hands of government, but then they insisted that the government follow their lead. Collectively, they presented a myriad of demands. But the overall pattern was to shake loose the existing relations between state and community and to alter the terms by which future relations would be negotiated. The activist phase altered the political conditions under which the entire field operated.

"DRUGS INTO BODIES"

To "rely solely on official institutions for our information," treatment activist John S. James wrote in 1986, "is a form of group suicide" (quoted in Epstein 1996, 195). Following such admonitions, community activists and patient advocates increasingly politicized scientific knowledge, challenging the authority of medical expertise in all aspects of HIV/AIDS epidemiology, treatment, and care, demanding, and receiving, access to policy- and decision-making procedures in the Food and Drug Administration (FDA), the Centers for Disease Control and Prevention (CDC), and the National Institutes of Health (NIH). Through the process of fighting these battles, the community activists redefined the standards for doctor-patient relations, engendering the notion of a patient-expert. They protested the invisibility of epidemiological practices, demanding that researchers present both their findings and their study designs to the public for review by patient advocates. They forced their way into clinical conferences, first as witnesses, then as presenters, and finally as "community representatives" on conference planning committees.

Community-based clinical research initiated the most involved partnership between community advocates and the public health sector. The notion of a community-directed program of monitored drug use and data collection began in 1984 with Mathilde Krim (later founder of the American Foundation for AIDS Research, or AmFAR); Michael Callen (a founding board member of People with AIDS Coalition of New York, or PWAC/NY); Joe Sonnabend, a physician with a large gay practice and connections to the Network and the Community Health Project (CHP); and activist Thomas Hannan. Callen, Sonnabend, and Hannan had all been founding organizers of the buyers' club PWA Health Group. The principal collaborators were community-based research advocates who set out to develop "the research arm of the people with AIDS Coalition" (Merton 1990, 502). In 1987, they formed a separate community-based organization (CBO) called the Community Research Initiative (CRI) to conduct their own trials. Founding member Max Navarre (1988, 145–46) described the origins of the group:

> Out of frustration with FDA foot-dragging on promising drugs for the treatment of AIDS and AIDS-related illnesses, the PWA Coalition developed the Community Research Initiative (CRI) to study these drugs in a community setting. Backed by a powerful and influential Institutional Review Board, utilizing the facilities of local physicians, and maintaining FDA-quality research, CRI seeks to achieve two goals: to give people access to the study of promising drugs that would otherwise be unavailable to them, and to prod the FDA into processing drugs that they might not otherwise explore.

Despite extensive resistance from the FDA and the National Institute on Allergies and Infectious Diseases (NIAID, which oversees clinical trials), CRI initiated and conducted the first successful clinical trial of an AIDS drug. Their data on aerosolized pentamadine, a PCP prophylaxis,[1] contributed significantly to its approval by the FDA (Arno and Feiden 1992; Harrington 1994) and changed the relationship between the world of researchers and that of patients (Merton 1990). This accomplishment led to recommendations from the Presidential Commission on the HIV Epidemic to integrate community research into the drug development process, which eventually led to the creation of the AIDS Clinical Trials Group (ACTG) (Arno and Feiden 1992, 118ff.).

The group's first success was also its greatest. Subsequent trials included some failures, some moderate successes, and some questions about data mismanagement. CRI reorganized in 1991 as the more stable AIDS Community Research Initiative of America (ACRIA) in the wake of financial and leadership crises. The group's newsletter, *ACRIA Update*, and its cosponsorship of several ongoing community forums placed it at the center of the "be your own expert" movement among people with HIV/AIDS. Virtually all of the treatment-involved CBOs reprinted CRI data for their members.

CRI sought to conduct studies that the government would be "embarrassed to spend money on," according to one physician-volunteer, a plan that produced variable results. Yet CRI's willful disregard for the business practices of scientific research was the principal benefit that they offered to the community. Founder Michael Callen, writing in 1989, described the AIDS national research policy as "passive genocide," according to CRI review board member Vanessa Merton. "It is difficult to overstate the intensity of the level of distrust and disdain many PWAs feel for the federal AIDS research effort" (Merton 1990, 532n2). CRI deliberately sought to both conduct a different kind of AIDS research and challenge the normative practices of medical research.

Community-based research was therefore pivotal in the emergence of treatment activism, the most conspicuous new path of community development. Treatment activists "challenged the formal procedures by which clinical trials are designed, conducted, and interpreted; confronted the vested interests of the pharmaceutical companies and the research establishment; demanded rapid access to scientific data; insisted on their right to assign priorities in AIDS research"; and drove the practices and priorities of community-based research (Epstein 1996, 32).

Most treatment activism was directed toward the fastest possible access to any and all drugs in development. ("Drugs into bodies" was an activist rallying cry.) For organizers, however, "access with answers" (a motto of the Treatment Action Group) joined questions of treatment access with an intense program of education on drug testing and development, the bureaucracy of clinical trials, and the politics of health funding. They campaigned for access to clinical trials—often the only source for new treatments—for women, people of color, and low-income people with HIV/AIDS. Later, treatment activists would become part of the review process for trial protocols, initiating a reevaluation of the use of placebos and double-blind studies with terminal patients and claiming for themselves the right to participate in trial design as advocates of patients-as-research-subjects. "There's no doubt that they've had an enormous effect," Stephen Epstein quotes former New York City health commissioner Stephen Joseph as saying. "We've basically changed the way we make drugs available" (Epstein 1996, 32).

DEVOTED SOLELY TO POLITICAL ACTION

ACT UP, the AIDS Coalition To Unleash Power, was not the first HIV/AIDS organization dedicated to street activism. The Gay and Lesbian Alliance against Defamation (GLAAD) formed in 1985 in response to the more blatantly homophobic media responses to HIV/AIDS, the rising numbers of gay men who had lost their jobs or their homes, and the increasing number of HIV-related political proposals to suspend various civil rights of homosexuals. Within the circles of AIDS organizing, both the Lavender Hill Mob, a GLAAD spin-off with membership ties to the New York AIDS Network, and the Silence=Death Project had begun staging "zaps" against public figures and wheat pasting the city with disturbing messages that criticized the gay community and its organizations for their quiescence about HIV/AIDS. ADAPT (the Association for Drug Abuse Prevention and Treatment) had planned the first civil disobedience to challenge syringe laws. The Testing the Limits Collective had begun documenting global "resistance" efforts. But

ACT UP absorbed the smaller HIV/AIDS protest efforts and gave rise to dozens of others. Almost from its first day, ACT UP became the organizational center of AIDS activism, averaging one demonstration every two weeks for about a year (Wolfe 1994, 222). Later renamed ACT UP/New York, as chapters sprang up in every city with significant HIV/AIDS rates in this country and elsewhere, ACT UP brought new levels of desperation and innovation to political activism around HIV/AIDS.

The formation, growth, and development of ACT UP integrated numerous strands of community organizing. Their commitment to outsider tactics shook up the alignments of the field of community-based HIV/AIDS work and spawned a new generation of groups and missions defined in relation to political activism. Relatively dormant now, ACT UP permanently altered the interorganizational relations of the organized community and enabled unprecedented new alliances between the state and the community. That they did so from a perspective of anger, and even hatred, mixed with physical threats, theatricality, and occasional sacrilege demonstrated the group's commitment to the process of change itself rather than to the construction of any specific new program. That task belonged to others working elsewhere in the field. As one informant explained, "ACT UP kicks the door down, then someone in a skirt or tie can go in and have a meeting." ACT UP had many successful campaigns on its own, but the lasting impact of the organization has been the effect it has had on the relationship between state agencies and the other CBOs.

Just prior to the formation of ACT UP in early 1987, as the Gay Men's Health Crisis (GMHC) sat solidly in the center of a growing web of AIDS service organizations (Chambré 1996), dissatisfaction with the lack of progress on other fronts had generated a heated discussion in the gay press and in community forums. Volunteers, caregivers, political organizers, and others debated the role of the community in relation to the state and the public health sector. Terms like *service* and *volunteer* and actions such as wearing red ribbons had taken on "the negative connotation of being empty gestures" according to an ACT UP volunteer who had designed the group's "You Can't Wear a Red Ribbon If You're Dead" poster campaign. In an example of what Paul Galatowitch (1999) has called "the failure of success," confidence in a public-private service partnership that had proven effective for less challenging health concerns had blunted the community's calls for sweeping changes. None of the largest and most influential CBOs in the field had the independence necessary to mount a serious campaign for reform against the few state agencies with which they routinely interacted. The pursuit of institutionally defined legitimacy had placed groups like GMHC at odds with many of its most dedicated supporters who valued their connection to "the community" above administrative practicality (Kayal 1993).

Recalling this period, Maxine Wolfe wrote that "it had become apparent to some members of the lesbian and gay community in New York that no matter how many service organizations we created, unless there were treatments available, all we could do was help people to die" (1994, 217). Wolfe and others advocated for new forms of organization to focus specifically on treatment and research. Then, in March 1987, at a community forum at the Lesbian and Gay Community Center, GMHC cofounder Larry Kramer challenged his audience to turn its frustration into a political force. His seemingly simple question, "Do we want to start a new organization devoted solely to political action?" resonated with an "already existing energy that [was] out there and help[ed] find a focus for its outlet" (Kramer 1989, 135, 137). Several organizational meetings quickly followed, and ACT UP was born.

ACT UP literally grew out of public discussion on the limitations inherent in the organized community's cooperative relationship with the state. Although the flow of money and information had improved considerably by the mid-1980s, the Reagan administration had given no indication that it shared the community's sense of urgency about HIV/AIDS. The organized community as a source of services and information gathering had a certain influence on HIV/AIDS policies, but it lacked power. ACT UP mobilized the potential power of the community against the state, which most active members considered negligent in combating HIV/AIDS (Elbaz 1992, 70). In its most prominent demonstrations, the organization seized offices at Burroughs-Wellcome in order to pressure the company into reducing the cost of AZT, shut down the stock exchange to protest "AIDS profiteering," and blocked access to the Food and Drug Administration's Rockville, Maryland, campus carrying "I died on placebo" placards to initiate changes in clinical trial design. At each event, they declared themselves with their signature motto "ACT UP, Fight Back, Fight AIDS," in which fighting back presumably declared their antithetical attitude toward the state, thereby breaking the pattern of state-community cooperation. "If we're not viewed as radical by the people in power, then they pay no attention," an ACT UP informant explained. "There has to be a degree of fear to be effective."

ACT UP defined itself from the start in contrast to GMHC and in opposition to the state. ACT UP was intended to be the real street activists, the voice of the community, not another bureaucracy serving the community. One informant who had initially joined ACT UP as "anger therapy" while working for GMHC eventually decided that GMHC had become a "big social service monstrosity" and felt that he could accomplish more within the ACT UP framework. For a time, many people worked with both organizations, wearing "different hats."

For the most part, these activists channeled their protest activities through ACT UP in addition to their ongoing work in GMHC and other AIDS service organizations. They did not seek to replace the community service perspective with the activism framework. Activist Mark Harrington referred to the service organizations and empowerment groups as "a foundation on which political agitation and treatment activism could be conducted" (Harrington 1994, 153). Ideologically, the new organization did not seek to supersede or undermine GMHC, but to introduce a new, nondestructive organizational form to the field of community-based AIDS work, free of the constraints inherent in the growing state-community partnership. For many, the ability to single-mindedly pursue protest actions within ACT UP allowed them to work more comfortably at their "day jobs" with the service organizations. Although there were evident personality conflicts enacted in ACT UP's formation (Kramer 1989), the groups still maintained a high degree of membership overlap. The formal organizational distinction between GMHC as the site of service and information dissemination working with the public health sector and ACT UP as the site of protest and policy demands working against it represented a new level of complexity in the division of labor within the organizational field of AIDS work. Operating outside of government institutions afforded the group the freedom to make the state the primary target of their actions, as many had wished.

Because ACT UP's mission was so large, seeking as they did to change people's lives locally and immediately while challenging both the state and pharmaceutical corporations nationally and while also upending the working relations between the organized community and government at all levels, ACT UP broke barriers between local actions and national politics. It was not surprising, therefore, that ACT UP should foster so many local chapters in so many cities, including, for a while, two in San Francisco. And because the group was so distinctly antagonistic to centers of (commercial and political) power, they did so without a federated structure. That is, the New York group was the first, the largest, and the most national of the chapters, but no one reported back to New York, and there was no national ACT UP leadership. Each group was its own entity.

ACT UP struggled to forge alliances with scientists while attacking research as a set of institutionalized practices, attending medical conferences as both presenters and protestors. Their activities spread across a wide range of protest and watchdog practices. They organized boycotts against drug companies whom they accused of profiteering and slowing the release of drugs, and doctors across the country actually initiated contact with ACT UP in order to join them (Elbaz 1992). Many of the activist organizations in New York whose missions are more specialized began as ACT UP committees. These splits, while not always friendly, seeded the HIV/AIDS activist community with seasoned organizers who shared many experiences and assumptions.

IS ACT UP AN ORGANIZATION?

ACT UP's name identified them as a "coalition" of individuals with shared interests or commitments. Their organizational structure was designed to be definitively loose and antiprofessional. It was a principle of the organizers that no one should have authority over anyone else. Meetings were facilitated by pairs of volunteers elected for six-month terms, three months out of phase with one another in order to discourage the formation of power blocs. There were no staff and no salaries. Much of the group's work was actually done in committees, working groups, and affinity groups. Affinity groups, which could be formed at any time by any subset of members who shared an interest, were independent entities in no way answerable to the rest of the membership. ACT UP's organizational structure encouraged members to act outside of the organizational structure.

In 1988, the organization adopted a set of pseudoformal procedures called "the working document" to give continuity to their organizational identity. "Now that this organization has an identity with the public and the press," the document states, "ACT UP is being called upon to articulate its policy or platform on certain issues in a formal manner" (ACT UP 1988:3). The document placed no limitations on what their positions would be or on who would write them, only that they would be approved by consensus. The organizational rules include specifications for terms of "office," limits on powers, and separate procedures for creating authorized and unauthorized zaps. Anyone can declare a zap—a rapidly organized protest event aimed at a specific target—at any meeting and can gather participants with or without approval from the membership. Since ACT UP rejects authority structures, there are separate procedures for carrying out protest actions that have been approved by the group and those that have been rejected by the group. There is no rule that says that the action should not take place, only that organizers cannot claim to represent the group as a whole, and that ACT UP doesn't have to cover the costs of unendorsed actions.

Unlike other CBOs, whose missions were often defined around a particular form of service or the needs of a particular community, ACT UP was defined around a confrontational political posture. Any member of the affected communities could, within that framework, pursue any issue. ACT UP's organization chart at the time of this research listed over fifty subgroups and committees, each with its own area of activism. The Latino Caucus smuggled AIDS drugs into Puerto Rico. The Treatment and Data Subcommittee shut down the Stock Exchange. The ACT UP Majority Actions Committee, so-named because of its focus on the non-White populations who were a majority among those with HIV, defined an AIDS reduction program incorporating realistic safer-sex education, harm reduction strategies, and the inclusion of straight men, people of color, and women in clinical trials (Elbaz 1992, 264). The Women's Caucus, which had begun in 1988 in response to *Cosmopolitan* magazine's claim that "women with 'healthy vaginas' would not contract HIV even if they had unprotected sex with an HIV-positive man" (Wolfe 1994, 231), organized a protest at the magazine's offices, called for a boycott of *Cosmo*, and produced an educational video about accurate HIV prevention information for women and about the proliferation of misinformation. Following these efforts, the Women's Caucus formed a research group, which published one of the first books dedicated to protecting women's health in the wake of HIV/AIDS (ACT UP Women's Handbook Group 1990).

Historically, ACT UP has had a flair for campiness that has attracted media attention. Dressing up during demonstrations and occasionally shouting slogans that have no meaning to anyone outside of the group is partly a reflection of their nonprofessionalism, but it is also essential to the ACT UP organizational form. It is an embrace of grassroots antiprofessionalism. They demonstrate that there are no restrictions placed on members' forms of expression, consistent with their claim that there should be no restrictions placed on their community's right to participate in decisions about their life and future. There is no formal process of judgment in ACT UP; this would validate rather than undermine the institutional authority system that rejects them.

The new activists did not focus on a new goal or a new thing to be done. They focused on new ways of doing things. Their underlying mission, to the extent that one can be identified, was to disrupt the routine practices of government and industry that had served people with HIV/AIDS so poorly. Their growth, in retrospect, was a logical response to the initial successes and stalled progress of the rest of the organized community. The field of HIV/AIDS groups prior to 1987 had done about as much as they could do as outsiders or minor allies to the public health sector. The existing organizations needed more involvement from the national health institutions and the various large research centers, public and private. It was in this context that ACT UP formed, not to solicit these institutions but to attack them. They adopted a carrot-and-stick approach in which ACT UP was the stick; later, someone else would have to find the carrot.

As outsiders to the state bureaucracy, ACT UP was structured for maximum embeddedness in its community of origin. The activists recognized that the community could only hope to shape the bureaucracy, not to replace it. Like the educators and service providers before them, ACT UP activists remained acutely conscious of their impact on the state's relationship with the community. Part of the struggle was to push the boundaries as far as possible before their own commitment to radical practice became self-destructive (Gamson 1995).

Yet, even as members remained committed to the notion that "everyone has to be heard," many activists eventually became frustrated with the long, disorganized meetings and stopped attending. Several key working groups and committees left the ACT UP organizational framework to pursue work in their areas of interest in a more pragmatic fashion. Such organizational splits spread the influence of ACT UP as a locus of collective identity, but they also removed effective leaders and active members from the group. By the mid-1990s, when many felt that "what's happening now in AIDS activism is working on the inside," the move back to GMHC or elsewhere became necessary. One of the first of these splits emerged from the work of treatment activists in the Treatment and Data Working Group.

ENEMIES: A LOVE STORY

"After ACT UP's successful FDA demonstration in October 1988, it needed to form a specialized subgroup, the Treatment+Data committee (T+D) to continue the research policy work as . . . activists began to become more integrated within research structures" (Harrington 1998). So recalled Mark Harrington, one of the original T+D activists whose work in treatment activism would eventually garner him a McArthur Fellowship. T+D began as a study group, poring through medical reports with the aid of textbooks and guest speakers. Since ACT UP prominently attacked the routine practices of clinical research, T+D sought to offer meaningful alternatives in terms that scientists could appreciate.

As one of its first projects, the T+D committee joined with the Actions Committee to begin a new affinity group to follow, critique, and change the AIDS Treatment and Evaluation Units (ATEUs) that coordinated clinical trials at that time. Jim Eigo took on the ATEU at New York University (NYU). In February 1989, he sent a letter to NYU identifying problems that the activists saw with the design and conduct of their trials and recommending changes that could make the unit more friendly to the needs of people with AIDS. "One of my suggestions in the letter: initiate what I called 'parallel trials,' that is, trials of experimental drugs that had only the loosest criteria and would run parallel to the drug's strictly limited phase two and three clinical trials designed to gather data for drug approval. . . . I sent a copy of this letter to Anthony Fauci, head of the NIH AIDS effort."

Parallel trials promised to solve three problems plaguing HIV/AIDS clinical research. First, the process of identifying, testing, approving, and distributing HIV medications took so long that advanced-stage patients were literally dying while waiting for new drugs. Patients were competing to get into trials under the assumption that untested but promising drugs represented their only opportunity for treatment. Second, researchers who adhered to strict scientific standards, including double-blind placebo trials followed by lengthy peer review prior to the release of their findings, were perceived by activists to be delaying the development of new drugs in the interests of their careers. The bench researchers involved with HIV/AIDS had little experience with clinical care and did not know how to deal with the blatant hostility and lack of cooperation they got from the people they saw as "trial subjects." And third, increasingly knowledgeable patients were already undermining the clinical trials. Community groups facilitated meetings among people in placebo trials wherein they would pool all of their medications and redistribute them, equalizing everyone's chances of getting some medication and completely invalidating all study data. Eigo's proposal provided a feasible technical solution to these known problems while also addressing the issues of public confidence.

In March of that year, Fauci, who was then the head of the OAR (Office of AIDS Research), came to New York to speak about AIDS research at the Institute of Medicine and to meet with ACT UP "on its home ground" (Arno and Feiden 1992, 173). Fauci introduced the concept of what he was then calling parallel track and got a positive response. T+D members pushed the idea further at the April International AIDS Conference in Montreal, including a poster session by Eigo. Here he adopted Fauci's language, thereby taking the stance of advocating in favor of the government position, even though he was actually pushing a community initiative of his own basic design. When Fauci formally introduced the concept in June at a treatment forum in San Francisco, activists on both coasts backed him completely, for a change. It was unclear who, if anyone, was changing sides. Back in Washington, D.C., where AIDS research coordinators at the FDA first heard about parallel track through the newspaper coverage of Fauci's comments, there was some resistance (Arno and Feiden 1992, 175). But both the proposal and its incorporation of community experts had entered into circulation in the HIV/AIDS research world. T+D claimed credit.

The T+D activists used civil disobedience and disruption to get their message across, but they also carefully rehearsed that message. With some exaggeration for effect, Larry Kramer credited their success to the discontinuity between their professional preparation and their activist demeanor. "Mark

[Harrington] would go in, and Jim [Eigo], too—they never took baths, and they smoked incessantly, and they looked like terrorists, but they opened their mouths and you couldn't believe the quality of the knowledge that came out" (*New Yorker* 1992, 40). Eigo's experiences epitomized the complexity of the activists' attempts to work both within and against the research bureaucracy. As he described it in an interview for this study,

> That summer I testified before a congressional subcommittee on the Parallel Track proposal, and I was asked to present a proposal for parallel track to an FDA Advisory Committee on which I'd be a guest member and have a vote. The committee voted in favor of the idea of Parallel Track, and voted to use my proposal as its rough draft. I was appointed to a Parallel Track Working Group of the National AIDS Program Office of the Department of Health and Human Services. . . . These were the first federal appointments for a grassroots AIDS activist. . . . During this time, I was arrested four times in AIDS-related civil disobedience and convicted once.

The Montreal Conference launched ACT UP's T+D group into the scientific policy arena, and they began to work the conference circuit to demand a place at the podium. Between the spring of 1989 and the San Francisco Conference in June 1990, activists and researchers actively forged what Robert Wachter, organizer of the 1990 conference, called "a fragile coalition" (Wachter 1991). Part of the activists' Montreal agenda had been community representation on what was now called the AIDS Clinical Trials Group (ACTG) (formerly the AIDS Treatment and Evaluation Units). Anthony Fauci had agreed, in principle, that they should be able to attend, but Fauci did not have the authority to make it happen. In October 1989, the ACTG investigators were scheduled to meet, and they chose not to invite the activists. Nonetheless, the activists came, and a portion of the conference time was forcibly redirected to the question of community participation. T+D accepted a compromise Community Constituency Working Group (CCWG), from which they could observe and comment on the scientific committees but not vote. They used this point of access to write a detailed and inflammatory insider's critique of the entire ACTG system, which Mark Harrington presented at the March 1990 ACTG meeting. Mutual hostilities and accusations increased. Again, participants struggled with the contradictions and fragility of the coalition. Activists demanded more participation while threatening to boycott future meetings. NIAID and the ACTG needed community cooperation, within the bounds of actually doing science. As described by Peter Arno and Karyn Feiden (1992, 230):

> Quite soon, Fauci got his chance to ask Harrington to stay [in the CCG]. . . . Peter Staley and Mark Harrington had called Fauci a few days earlier, told him

they planned to be on the NIH campus and suggested an informal dinner. Fauci made the social arrangements, and when they arrived for dinner that evening, he greeted them warmly.

"What brings you down here?" he asked. Harrington answered candidly. "We're taking pictures of the NIH campus for a demonstration in May."

Both the activists and the research policy leaders hoped to come to terms by the June International AIDS Conference. The conference opened with considerable representation from both activists and police. Wachter's description of the 1990 conference focused mostly on the negotiations for a working relationship between the two sides that would neither force scientists to give up their meeting to the activists nor require ACT UP to stand down. Wachter was keenly aware of the dual role that the activists had defined for themselves, a role that made him both ally and enemy. While the conference hall swelled with uninvited participants, including an unknown number of activists with forged press passes poised to disrupt, several prominent activists contributed to the opening session as invited speakers.

Next on the videotape was Larry Kramer, filmed as he stood in the sunshine of New York's Central Park. On his T-shirt was a quote—"By Any Means Necessary"—from black radical Malcolm X. . . . Many reluctant whites dealt eagerly with [Martin Luther] King, the theory goes, because they feared that they might have to confront Malcolm X if they did not. Perhaps this was Larry Kramer's agenda. (Wachter 1991, 200–201)

THE CO-OPTATION PROBLEM

Having significantly influenced the agenda and with several opportunities to address the assembly as invited guests, ACT UP reserved its more disruptive activities for a few key targets. For the most part, activists and researchers emphasized their common interests. This collaboration between community activists and government researchers was an accomplishment of community organizing, but the activists' deference to the treatment specialists also threatened to co-opt ACT UP's primary source of power. Further compromises during subsequent events brought the issue to the foreground, and it became a matter of debate. Even successful demonstrations raised the specter of co-optation. As one activist shouted out from the floor following the report on a peaceful demonstration in Washington, D.C., "Since when do we make deals with cops?" The stage was set for either an organizational innovation or an organizational catastrophe.

The international conference had provided new opportunities for conflict, additional concessions to the activists, and new scientific data that were almost completely overlooked in the wake of the political conflicts and negotiations. ACT UP's T+D group had gained considerable ground as they acquired the right to participate in review panels, clinical-trial design committees, and policy planning strategies. But they did not participate as clinical experts; they participated alongside clinical experts. Their role was that of community representatives. "Even if researchers were dubious about the patient community's ability to gauge what research was most important, they certainly recognized the practical values of cooperation and negotiation in order to ensure accrual. In this sense, a basic 'credibility achievement' of treatment activists has been their capacity to present themselves as the legitimate, organized voice of the people with AIDS or HIV infection (or, more specifically, the current or potential clinical trial subject population)" (Epstein 1996, 252).

Through their expertise and their selective targeting, the T+D activists found their access to the policy domain increasing. At that time, however, they were working from within an organizational framework that sought to represent all of the people threatened by HIV/AIDS, on all political matters. The access that the group was offered was clearly limited to certain forums where a small group of activists had achieved proficiency in the language and technology that was already in place, and where issues of gender, class, and routine discrimination would remain secondary to the long-term research agenda. It was also based on the premise that the activists would participate in an existing system of policy making on the state's own terms. For ACT UP, the new insider access was the opportunity to gain concessions in one arena in exchange for a reduction of efforts in all others, which amounted to a form of organizational, and possibly political, suicide.

Stephen Epstein (1996) related that the "men" behind T+D sought to develop the new partnership with the state health policy sector. However, not all branches of AIDS activism sought such accommodation with the state, whether the opportunity existed or not. Members of ACT UP's T+D group recalled that an "element" of ACT UP who felt that "you should never be on the inside" became quite "antagonistic" to the new form of work. Many in ACT UP feared, realistically, that the organization would lose its unique position if it got too "cozy" with the state. The Women's Action Committee, in particular, felt that the growing focus on treatment work was damaging the rest of the organization's mission, and they proposed a six-month moratorium on direct contact with the government. T+D adamantly opposed this. The moratorium, in keeping with the principles of the organization, would have committed the treatment activists to a policy of outsider agitation rather than the new insider tactics at which they were becoming experts.

One informant recalled this period as a particularly existential crisis. Over the course of several weeks, the group endured an "acrimonious debate" concerning its identity and public role, with no emerging proposal on which to vote. The deadlock was broken when members of T+D independently proposed that they would leave ACT UP to form a new organization. Late in 1991, core members of the T+D group split from ACT UP to form TAG, the Treatment Action Group. Although it had taken time to recognize it, the organization had come to occupy two distinct niches within their field, and they needed to split them apart in order to protect the integrity and independence of both. Many members of both organizations perceived the split as both a fracture and a strategic division of labor. Informants concur that although the two organizations were able to collaborate following the split, there were individuals who were unable to bridge that gap. One TAG member, describing the role of ACT UP as the perennial "bad cop," defined the new organization as a necessary compliment to it. "TAG can be considered a good cop by the medical research establishment, but a bad cop by the pharmaceutical industry. . . . The important point is to be aware of the value of these roles and to be willing to use them towards a given purpose."

TAG's mission was defined in general terms around the treatment needs of all people living with HIV, present and future. TAG took on multiple roles, both meeting with government officials and organizing acts of civil disobedience. In the case of civil disobedience, "organizing" frequently meant trying to get ACT UP to mobilize its members. "They have the numbers," a TAG member explained. As treatment specialists, TAG sought collaborations with medical professionals. Members held numerous community advisory seats on NIH panels and routinely reviewed clinical trial protocols before they were submitted to the FDA. As part of the activist network, they were prepared to disrupt these panels or undermine subsequent policy recommendations if they did not feel that the interests of their community were being served. As experts, they brought their messages to the sites of clinical research—attending virology meetings, AIDS conferences, and visiting research campuses, invited or otherwise. Yet, as community representatives, they also brought their charts and tables to neighborhood forums where current clinical data are hard to come by and where such expertise was viewed with suspicion.

TAG's presence outside of state and activist communities often forced both sides to accept compromises, at the risk of alienating everyone. TAG's role was curious, since they were known by the people with whom they interacted as former outsiders who were now working on the inside. In a sense, they chose to emphasize their collaborations with research over their community location, but ultimately they formed a new bridge between the two. TAG had to move through different locations in the field before finding what one board member called their "unusual niche." Almost as professional as GMHC, and not quite as angry as ACT UP, TAG could only define themselves in an environment that already supported the two extremes. They made themselves the activists who were willing to negotiate, freeing ACT UP/NY from having to do so and thereby reinforcing ACT UP's uncompromising stance. Responding to TAG's mediating stance, agencies of the public health sector used them as the point of entry to the community, a contact that was able to minimize the contention that accompanied each new study proposal.

GMHC might have been the most successful policy and money insiders, but TAG formed a link with the NIH through which the state negotiated with the community. This was a role that GMHC could not have sought. Their relations with the state were already too established; GMHC was a good supplicant and the state a good provider. The treatment activists, who often met NIH institute heads for dinners and other social occasions, had, as members of ACT UP/NY's T+D group, previously burned more than one of these directors in effigy. As a TAG member once observed, "Only Nixon could go to China."

ACT UP, as a site of community activism, had brought together members of the affected communities to speak and act in their own voice. TAG, as indigenous clinical experts and appointed community representatives, spoke on behalf of the community within policy debates that occurred outside of the community. They spoke to health officials in the language of health officials. With no clearly identifiable constituency, TAG had little to do with community mobilization efforts, concentrating their efforts on gaining voice in debates on research strategies, federal appropriations, and technical oversight. Summarizing the treatment activists' campaign for NIH reform, which began at the Montreal conference and ended with legislation authorizing the formation of an Office of AIDS Research, Mark Harrington observed that "in just five years, we had gone from acts of civil disobedience to acts of Congress" (Harrington 1998). Indirectly, Harrington was answering the ACT UP critique of TAG's insider political posture. "Our job is not to be invited to coffee or to shmooze at a cocktail party," Maxine Wolfe said the year before in her history of the same events. "Our job is to make change happen as fast as possible, and direct action works for that. . . . Without an 'outside,' an 'inside' is just politics as usual" (Wolfe 1997).

TAG had the opportunity to occupy a mediating location, blurring the boundary between inside and outside. Within research and policy arenas, they could speak legitimately as community representatives without actually organizing a constituency or tarnishing their personal connections through protest or threats. On occasion, however, TAG members have handed their insider information over to their colleagues at ACT UP/NY and have quietly watched as the "outsiders" brought pressure to bear. In one 1994 meeting, while a group member reported that the FDA still refused to look into an underground clinical trial that TAG was endorsing, others suggested finding someone else further outside the political arena to pursue the fight. "You mean an underground underground?" the presenter asked. TAG had become, in effect, an aboveground underground, which took the edge off its coercive influence but increased its access.

The debates preceding the formation of both ACT UP and TAG provide explicit examples of community concerns, just as the launching of each group demonstrated the use of diversification as a solution. In both cases, organizers wished to expand their work into new areas using different tactics, but they feared that the new approach would compromise the benefits of their ongoing work. In both cases, community organizers were able to pursue both goals by expanding the field of organizations into new areas. This multiorganizational process provided some degree of protection to community autonomy while allowing them to form necessary connections with state agencies. By providing multiple organizational forms within the same domain of action, the CBOs were able to represent their communities of origin, often against the interests of the state, without fostering an entirely hostile pattern of interaction. Such strategies have been examined before, including "the radical flank effect" (Haines 1984) observed in the civil rights movement.

If, however, the flexibility of the community gave them greater influence in their dealings with the state, then it would follow that the state would wish to establish some regularity in its relations with the organized HIV/AIDS community. This is indeed what occurred in the early 1990s. As the state formalized the terms of subsequent state-community relations, the community had to choose between rejecting the participation and support that they had long sought and working strictly on the government's terms. With little hesitation, the community accepted the state's deal. Chapter 6 will examine this transition, which effectively replaced the urban action network form with a system of block grants to service consortia.

NOTE

1. *Pneumocystis* pneumonia (PCP), one of the defining characteristics of late-stage HIV disease, is a frequent cause of death among people with HIV/AIDS.

Chapter Six

A New State-Centered Strategy

Community-based organizing defined the contours of HIV/AIDS work. They set the priorities, challenged policy, forged new alliances, and mobilized "outsider" pressure tactics in order to penetrate the structures of the state AIDS policy domain. Community-based collective actors defined what living with HIV/AIDS meant, measured the needs of people living with HIV/AIDS, and defined the responses in education, prevention, care, and even treatment research. They did not simply fill the gaps in community care in areas where the government had been slow to act. Community-based organizations provided those government researchers and policy planners who were active in HIV/AIDS work with the contacts and resources they needed to do their jobs in areas where the government had not acted.

The active, vocal, and aggressive network of community-based action that organizers created in New York City may have provided people living with HIV/AIDS with a strong political presence, but it could not begin to cover the basic health and social service needs of more than one million affected people throughout the country. The empowerment movement could only directly reach those who had communities to join. Beyond that, the community needed the state. It was inevitable that the organized community would recede in influence when the state chose to come forward. The lasting accomplishment of the organized community was to give shape to the organizational field of HIV/AIDS work before the state took it over. That occurred in the early 1990s.

MULTIPLE NETWORK MODELS

Eventually, the federal government had to define its own HIV/AIDS agenda. When it did so, it imported most of the major assumptions of the community-based mobilization. But politically, it could not simply begin to support the community network with which it had been fighting for nearly ten years. Having denounced the activists and educators as pornographers and anarchists, state agencies were probably not in a comfortable position to hire the same people to manage the system that they would build. They needed a different, centrally controlled model to supplant the community network. Such a model was incompatible with the New York City network. But one like it had been thriving in San Francisco.

The New York and San Francisco models differed most significantly in two key areas: scope and structure. Whereas the New York model grew increasingly diverse while remaining decentralized, the San Francisco networks were both centralized and oriented around service provision. This process promoted necessary services as defined by community groups while simultaneously limiting the role and the voice of the organized community in the HIV/AIDS policy domain. In San Francisco, where the organized gay community had routine access to government and the public health sector, it was natural that the city and state would consult the community before implementing an HIV/AIDS response. That question had been resolved already in past battles. In New York, which had become the central point in AIDS-related activism nationally and globally, the transition to a government-centered HIV/AIDS policy meant reducing community organizations from the array of activism, advocacy, research, and auditing functions to an advisory role.

The new state-community relationship guaranteed state support for most of what the community had been doing on its own, other than politics, with the understanding that the dynamic and unpredictable system of defining new needs and pressing new claims would be funneled through fixed channels and predefined points of control. Whereas previously, organizations working in different areas had been able to promote the perspectives that emerged from their work by reshuffling priorities and calling forth new spheres of activity, the new state-centered system of relations began with a fixed set of priorities, set tasks, and a consistent language. It adopted the terms and definitions with which the community had been working, but it did so in a way that reified those definitions. The state approach placed primary responsibility for care, services, and education on private nonprofit organizations while retaining regulatory authority for itself in exchange for which it also provided funding. Any nonprofit organizations that wanted to participate in this system would have to accept this single perspective. But the money was certainly good, so most of them did.

THE CONSORTIA MODEL

When the federal government set out to define its own HIV/AIDS agenda, it recognized that "contact with the most affected groups is required" (Altman 1988, 302). The principal mechanism for this contact and coordination has been the federal Ryan White Comprehensive AIDS Resources Emergency (CARE) Act of 1990. The programs funded under this act are not the only federal source of community support for HIV/AIDS work, but the CARE Act provides the largest, longest-running, and most broadly defined government-based system of community support. The Ryan White CARE Act, named for the country's most prominent "innocent victim" of HIV/AIDS, defined a model for community-based provision of care and services that replaced the complex, informal interorganizational relations of the network of nonprofits with isolated, formally defined consortia. This model of public-private partnership derived from the experiences of the Robert Wood Johnson AIDS Health Services Program, which had actually sought to emulate the more cooperative relationship between local government and community in San Francisco.

The accomplishments of the organized community in New York were all the more remarkable and necessary due to their isolation. The other epicenter, San Francisco, was a very different story. (For details on that story, see Arno 1986; Shilts 1987; and Stoller 1998.) "During the first decade of the AIDS epidemic, the United States produced the very best policy—and the very worst," public policy analysts Donald Kirp and Ron Bayer wrote in 1992. "The best was what came to be represented as the San Francisco model. The model . . . included private care-giving, with everything from emotional counseling and cooked meals to pet care provided for people with AIDS by organizations largely staffed with volunteers and partly subsidized by government" (Kirp and Bayer 1992, 361). Mervyn Silverman, former director of San Francisco's Department of Health, called it a "coordinated community response," in which, for the most part, the community responded and the health department coordinated. "Rather than expect the community alone to plan, initiate, and implement all AIDS programs, however, we began, in San Francisco, with the idea of a cooperative and collaborative arrangement—in essence, a partnership—between government and community groups. We looked at the situation as a new type of health crisis that needed a new approach" (Silverman 1987, 171). Community organizers in San Francisco had begun with the same expectations and approaches as the New York groups. Both looked to health officials for leadership. In San Francisco, they found it.

As early as 1985, the Robert Wood Johnson Foundation (RWJF), a leading supporter of health care and policy analysis, began to investigate ways in which they could have an impact on the medical and social needs for people living with HIV/AIDS. In conjunction with health policy analysts, city health officials, the Health Resources and Services Administration (HRSA), and the San Francisco Department of Health, RWJF began the AIDS Health Services Program (AHSP), which funded its first demonstration sites in 1986 (HRSA 2004). The intent of these demonstration projects, in addition to improving care and services for people living with HIV/AIDS, was to introduce the San Francisco model to other cities throughout the country (Mor et al. 1994, 7). Fortunately, RWJF also funded a series of evaluations and assessments, leading to a plethora of publications on the progress of these projects in the intervening years. The summary that follows derives from the published AHSP and CARE Act evaluations.

The RWJF projects followed the "care coordination" criteria now mandated for those metropolitan areas receiving Ryan White Comprehensive AIDS Resources Emergency Title I and Title II funding (hereafter, CARE). The original demonstration project was established "in response to the perceived inadequacy of appropriate medical care and community-based services for persons with AIDS" (Allen et al. 1995, 48). "Although community-based HIV services are essential, there are serious gaps in these programs," noted Susan Penner (1995, 218), whose work was independent of the RWJF evaluations. V. Mor and colleagues use the term "maximizing system responsiveness to the AIDS crisis" (1994, 8), which refers to the efficient allocation of resources, addressing the concern for duplication of services and other organizational inefficiencies, possibly ahead of the desire for maximum coverage of needs. Consortia arrangements brought CBOs into routine and formal contact with hospitals, hospices, and local services for housing, mental illness, and other factors beyond the scope of the HIV/AIDS community's expertise. Such alliances have also been described as "forced marriages" (Fleishman et al. 1992, 560). The ability of organizations in the consortia to work together was variable in all of the evaluation studies, often due to power struggles and a lack of trust as well as a lack of consensus over the goals and tasks of the consortia members. In much of the country, the most difficult task was initiating enough community-based work to encompass the full range of necessary services. In New York, where there were more than enough groups already, the consortia had the effect of replacing the dynamic interorganizational relations of the community with a hierarchical system of coordination, reducing the input of active community nonprofits.

Among other requirements, the consortia were mandated to establish "planning councils [that were] 'broadly representative' of HIV service providers, community leaders, persons infected and affected by HIV, and state government" (McKinney 1993, 115). Consortia were also required (in the initial program plan) to select an incorporated "lead agency" to receive the grant and to oversee the money management. Many community-based organizations were unaccustomed to such an emphasis on accountability. Whether they considered the requirements intrusive or helpful, few of the community organizations were prepared to take on the bureaucratic burden of coordinating the new consortia. One study found that while community groups were sometimes reluctant to surrender some of their autonomy to state agencies, state health departments were generally perceived as the most legitimate consortia leaders (Fleishman et al. 1992).

Structural characteristics varied considerably throughout the AHSP sites and their offshoots, depending on such issues as the number of participants and the role of the state health departments in the consortia (Mor et al. 1994, 58–63). In one study of consortia across six states, established AIDS service organizations (ASOs) were defined as lead agencies in three cases. In two cases, agencies were chosen by consortia to act as fiscal managers without additional authority. In the remaining case, the participants incorporated the entire consortium as a 501(c)(3) nonprofit service organization and were able to manage the grant as a group (McKinney 1993, 119).[1] In two of the consortia led by service organizations, "members expressed uncertainty about what the consortia is supposed to do and how its role differs from that of the ASO" (121).

Authority relations were a frequent problem, and the consortia often had difficulties negotiating their collective purpose and fixing boundaries around the roles of each participant group. Reliance on a lead agency provided several important functions that reflected the premises of the funding agencies over the priorities of the CBOs. First, although the consortia were composed primarily of community agencies, the emphasis on an acceptable lead group created incentives for a least one major service provider in each network to emulate a government service agency. Furthermore, defining that agency as the "lead" group, or indeed requiring each community consortium to identify their own lead group, gave the state and other regulators a single point of contact that would speak their language and possibly share their values. Defining a single lead agency as a service organization with a broad mandate also meant that advocacy issues and minority agendas would be minimized in the overall workings of the community-based interorganizational structure while potentially still remaining somewhere in the consortia. Groups that were primarily concerned with, for example, political voice or even access to treatment for people of color would have to negotiate those priorities with the consortium prior to taking them up with the state or the media. Finally, giving fiscal authority to a single community-based corporation addressed fears that the community groups would have too many interests and too many voices to get the job done in a consistent and reliable manner. It also buffered some of the smaller groups from the pressures of accounting and oversight. The structure created an implicit hierarchy of goals, crowned by service provision.

Mandated cooperatives were specifically designed to provide a division of labor with as little redundancy as possible. An interim goal for a consortium in formation was to "regularize" their activities. Drawing on their experience and knowledge of community resources and needs, consortium members were expected to define a set of goals and procedures for achieving them and then commit to formalizing the procedures. By definition, consortium participants were expected to develop their ability to anticipate client needs, secure resources, and deliver services to meet those needs. This mandated goal, manifestly practical, had the latent effect of undermining the prospects for political representation. "Voluntary consortia often were founded for political advocacy and legislative lobbying and to exert influence on public policies affecting HIV agencies and their clients," Penner observed. "By contrast, mandated consortia are expected to allow the mandating agency, usually a government authority or funder, to exert control over the members" (1995, 222). One cannot advocate, let alone disrupt, from within such a framework. "Unfortunately for the intentions of many AIDS CBOs, it proved to be difficult to provide both individualized care (providing services) and system advocacy within the same organization, particularly with the addition of case management to an agency's repertoire of services" (Allen et al. 1995, 54).

Although most of the evaluation studies noted the conflict in organizational missions and the shift in focus among CBOs that resulted, none of them actually identified the consortia requirements as the cause. Rather, the reports tended to suggest that the multiple functions previously pursued by so many groups were merely inconsistent with one another and that simplification was inevitable. With reference to Weberian routinization and the "institutionalization phase" of an organization's "life cycle," for example, S. Allen and colleagues attributed the mission creep to a seemingly natural progression, of which the consortia demands were but one contributing factor. The effect was therefore not part of the formal evaluations of the consortia.

The purpose of the consortia was to provide necessary care and services, not representation, and program evaluators worked with those assumptions. The evaluations focused on the consortia's abilities to implement the desired changes rather than on the desirability of the reorganization. Thus, consortia were often found to be dysfunctional if the participant groups could not agree to a new hierarchy and successful if they were able to function under one. Following this approach, Mor and colleagues found that the perceived quality and "legitimacy" of the lead agencies was one of the best predictors of consortium functioning, with state health departments generally achieving the highest legitimacy evaluations (1994, 67). Overall, state agencies had the most reliable funding and the smoothest functioning, despite high bureaucratic overhead, while community-based nonprofits achieved a much higher standing in the perceptions of the communities in which they worked. McKinney (1994) notes that among CBOs, AIDS service organizations had the most experience with the kinds of tasks, both in terms of service delivery and acquiring revenue, that were central to the operation of an AIDS service consortium.

Informants in New York have suggested that, with time and experience, state reviewers "relaxed" the requirements concerning lead agencies, at least within New York City, and allowed CBOs more leeway to manage their own interorganizational relations. Although there have been no studies of the changing role of the lead agencies, the study by Fleishman and colleagues (1992) of "lead agency identity" predicted that there would be difficulties with this design. In most AHSP sites, the lead agency was selected after the consortium had been fully established, and it limited its special functions to fiscal and administrative ones. The CARE Act language suggested a more encompassing role that would limit the community's participation in the definition of consortia identities, reducing their attractiveness to established groups and constraining their flexibility.

Mor and colleagues also reported that AHSP consortia were funded in part to help mobilize communities of affected people. They were therefore a potential means for empowerment in communities that had not organized on their own, although the consortia did not encourage community participation outside the arenas of health care and social services. "In addition," they suggested, "a consortium can serve as a symbolic reminder of the commitment to solve a community-wide problem" (Mor et al. 1994, 65–66). As the demographics of HIV/AIDS shifted away from the demographic base of the most established service organizations—as HIV rates among people of color, especially women of color, overtook rates among White men—consortia organizers mandated "representation" of communities of color on the planning boards and in decision-making positions (Allen et al. 1995). Consortium expansion into minority communities represented commitment, symbolically, where the existing community commitment had been judged insufficient or otherwise incompatible with consortia goals. Even so, a 1996 evaluation of "Women and the CARE Act" in eight metropolitan areas found that women as well as both women and men of color, consistently found barriers to participation in Ryan

White Planning Councils, with the result that funding priorities often failed to take into account the needs of most people with HIV (Center for Women Policy Studies 1996).

The consortia needed to reach out to a broader range of CBOs. The service networks required non-White organizations but not necessarily as equal partners. The applicant groups still had to apply through the lead agencies, the perceived "White" groups, for their share of the funding. The AHSP and its successors thus contributed both money and legitimacy in areas where volunteer-based work and public contributions were perceived to have been unable to establish a caregiving system, simultaneously creating both a support system and a dependency/authority relationship. Martha McKinney's study of a sample of consortia indicated that most community-based member organizations were gay centered, and participation by people of color and their representative organizations was redefined as an "outreach" problem. "Although people of color were underrepresented in five consortia, only one consortium had made a vigorous effort to increase minority participation." The one exception adopted its outreach efforts after the local health department had required a more diverse membership as a condition of continued funding (McKinney 1993, 118). In what might serve as a synopsis for the service model nationwide, the author concluded that the consortia she had studied were generally hampered by mixed messages and a particular lack of clarity about "who the members represent" (119).

In areas where a substantial community mobilization had already occurred, "a more ambitious goal for a service delivery consortium [was] to reduce the fragmentation and discontinuity in the delivery system itself. To achieve this goal require[d] altering the pattern or nature of interorganizational relations" (Mor et al. 1994, 66). Consortia sought to do considerably more than facilitate new relationships. They altered the nature of the interorganizational relations already in place, where they existed. They sought to bring communities out of the supposedly haphazard realm of homegrown remedies and self-help and firmly into a social service model of living assistance. This change, from the existing and hard-to-evaluate combination of political, medical, and service-oriented community-based work into a model of integrated services, was described by organizers as a political act and a form of empowerment. The consortia were intended to empower communities by providing a formalized, although singular, point of access to the domain of health policy.

Community-based nonprofits in New York and elsewhere voluntarily entered into the new arrangements, but not without difficulty and some renegotiation of terms. Despite the relative lack of formal authority relationships and reports of reasonable autonomy among consortium partners, at least in areas like San Francisco where HIV/AIDS community groups had already been established (Penner 1995), participating CBOs faced increasing service demands and limited funding, straining their ability to deliver on their obligations to clients. Organizational resources were channeled into a social service model with little flexibility, high accountability, and almost no remaining discretionary funds for other interests. Many of the CBOs, including the New York groups examined here, had been heavily invested in boundary-spanning activities. Evaluators found that under the terms of the new service contracts boundaries became firmer, and formal linkage agreements replaced anything that resembled "redundant" efforts. Yet in New York, the specific requirements of CARE Act funding explicitly redirected community networks from existing informal systems of coordination into formal authority structures. Indeed, that outcome appears to have been built into the support model and backed by contract. One Texas evaluation explicitly noted that "control of HIV/AIDS service dollars and programmatic decisions was shifted away from the traditional AIDS agencies and their supporters in the gay community and taken over by the professional welfare bureaucracy and county elected officials. . . . The largely conservative body sought to distance itself from AIDS-related controversy by appointing a governing body for AIDS programs . . . that reflected both its desire for strong fiscal management and a rejection of outspoken political advocacy" (Bielefeld and Scotch 1996, 49). As Penner observed, "Domain consensus, defined as agreement among organizations regarding roles and tasks, is less problematic if interorganizational relations are mandated rather than voluntary" (1995, 221). If the organizations cannot agree among themselves to adopt the funding agency's priorities, then it can become a condition for ongoing support.

Funders impose restrictions. Whether they are protecting their investments against waste and mismanagement or explicitly seeking to influence the outcomes of the work they fund, those who control "the purse strings" expect more than results. They expect to have influence in the process. When the funder is the state, there are ideological restrictions as well as protections against the influence of ideology. But there are also patterns and habits that give shape to what government agencies treat as the best practices, those worthy of support. Chao Guo and Muhittin Acar (2005, 347) identify "two competing influences" that tend to result "from reliance on government funding: first, the pressure toward formalized collaboration is likely to increase as an organization receives government funding; second, the deterrent from funding requirements actually increases with the diversity of government funding streams." That is, government agencies prefer formal and measurable (and perhaps regulated) collaborations over informal ones. But each agency and funding stream is relatively independent and is likely to have its own criteria, its own demands, and its own reporting procedures. Thus, an organization that secures a mix of funding from multiple government agencies is discouraged from managing too many links and collaborations since they all have to be explained and justified in different ways and since some might meet one grant's criteria while threatening another. A nonprofit recipient of public funds can limit this problem by being equally compartmentalized in its own work, which reduces the use of its interorganizational networks. Interestingly, groups that are primarily funded by a single government source, as is the case for CARE Act grantees, have more flexibility. However they choose to approach the funding restrictions, there is only one set of rules.

Outside contracts, while vital to such practical goals as the expansion of services, pressure organizations to maintain development offices to review requests for proposals, to prepare applications, and to train staff in grant writing. Again in Weberian terms, organizations shifted resources from their ostensible missions to their own maintenance and expansion as they formalized their operations. But whereas Max Weber wrote about the internal motivations of organizational leaders to protect their groups' continuity (Weber 1978 [1922]), the principal impetus for restructuring in the HIV/AIDS field came from external requirements (cf. DiMaggio and Powell 1983). Organizations seeking contracts had to demonstrate their ability to maintain a viable organizational infrastructure. They also faced pressures to alter their operating processes away from those favored by the groups' communities toward those favored by funding agencies. Organizations seeking formal support also had to demonstrate their ability to maintain linkages. That need, ironically, devalued the uncountable number of informal interconnections running among all of the community-based organizations in the HIV/AIDS field in New York and gave priority to formal linkage agreements.

The Competitive Aspect

CARE Act support was based on the logic of block grants. One of the ways in which the program sought to ensure efficient collaboration to avoid redundant investment was to channel funding only through the consortia, typically at a level that was lower than the sum of the support required by individual consortium members to provide the same functions. The various linked groups with overlapping missions had to either reapportion their clients by geographic or demographic characteristics, or fight it out among themselves. Allen and colleagues noted that funding requirements that tied allocation to development work with CBOs organized by people of color "result[ed] in increased competition among agencies for slices of the resource pie and considerable debate around 'ownership' of the issues" (Allen et al. 1995, 55). One of the functions of the lead agency, then, was to arbitrate these disputes.

The smaller CBOs could only receive steady funding after it was filtered through the larger ones, who themselves were encouraged to define, as a billable service, their ability to facilitate the transfer as efficiently as possible. The smaller CBOs, who might previously have enjoyed no funding at all from the established groups, were thus brought into a clientalistic relationship with those CBOs that were "successful in establishing working relationships with . . . the local health departments" (Allen et al. 1995, 48).

The "clientalistic" relationship among the lead agencies—defined in part according to their "standing" in the larger community—and the less secure agencies that must apply for support or participation problematizes the issues of representativeness. This difficulty was actually found to be greater when the lead agencies came from the community rather than from the government. State support for and involvement in community-based work creates "a tension . . . within the rank and file . . . who feel estranged from the new bureaucrats their own movement seems to have spawned" (Altman 1988, 310). A single organization that tries to maintain strong ties to both government and its community risks alienating both.

Organization and Environment

Ann Dill, a colleague of the authors of the Brown University AHSP evaluation (Mor et al. 1994), undertook an institutional analysis of four of the consortia in the Brown study. Quickly reaffirming the major findings of past evaluations, Dill attempted to explain the degree of success or failure in interorganizational coordination by examining the lead agencies, the coordinating structures, and the institutional environments in which they were established.

The most successful case occurred in Dallas, where "a loose coalition of agencies, basically the membership of the coordinating committee which was a once-a-month get together to talk about what we were all doing [informant description]" started to look into the grant (Dill 1994). They were unable to reach any sort of consensus about how to restructure themselves in accordance with the grant guidelines. So one of the decisions they made was to identify an outside agency, a "neutral" party with administrative capacity, to serve as their "lead agency."

The Dallas agencies had a coordinating structure of sorts already. Each group did what it did, and they had representatives who met regularly. The exchanges were voluntary and created a dense network of links from just about everyone to everyone else through this coordinating body. By enrolling the support of an outside agency, they were choosing, by consensus, to weaken the consensus model of decision making. They ceded a degree of authority to another agency in exchange for (1) the agreement that the lead agency would carry most of the burden of administration for the consortia, leaving the individual groups to focus on the services that they already provided and (2) the opportunity to receive AHSP funding. "The neutrality of the [lead agency] was reinforced by the fact that the individual who took the lead in developing the proposal, and who subsequently became the project director, had no prior involvement with AIDS; the reaction to this by the other agencies was described by this person as being 'Thank God he didn't bring any turf with him'" (Dill 1994, 356).

In Atlanta, the lead agency was a prominent community-based AIDS service organization that had been fairly successful on its own. It was given the leadership role by consensus, with the group's director thereby becoming the leader of the consortia. Once in this role, the group "faced considerable organizational instability. Its first director, an individual experienced mainly with gay advocacy groups, proved unsatisfactory as an administrator; the second, more bureaucratically oriented, was seen as too officious. Both resigned under pressure from the board of directors" (Dill 1994, 359). The agency and its third director had legitimacy in the nonprofit sector and in the HIV/AIDS field. But the consortia had further operational difficulties due to their lack of legitimacy in the institutional domain of health care services. That is, the hospitals and public health agencies treated the consortium as a client, not a partner. There were incidents of hostility, political competition, and a general reluctance to share information. Neither the researcher nor her informants felt that the overall program was very successful due to the limited nature of the community's integration into the existing institutional framework.

Dill's third case, Miami, had a number of existing agencies that could participate in a consortium, but the target communities were fragmented, not well organized themselves, and not networked. The first challenge of the grant applicants was therefore to bring the community groups into any organized structure at all. The lead agency, a hospital, had to convince the community groups of its legitimacy and then constantly pressure the organizations into participating in the continuum of care exchanges required by the consortium. They were able to channel needed resources into communities of need and to foster the growth of community-based support. On the other hand, the relationship between the lead agency and the participating AIDS service organizations was often formal and contractual rather than cooperative or flexible.

Dill concludes, convincingly, that the differences among the cases demonstrate that organizational forms differ according to the demands and expectations of the institutional environments, particularly along a continuum from the most normative to the most technical. Where trust and legitimacy are high and required, interorganizational relations are often characterized by loose coupling (each agent having a fair amount of autonomy), informal communication, and reciprocity. That's the normative case. If goals are defined in terms of technical deliverables, then top-down control, monitoring, and contract disputes dominate. Yet, most interesting of all, since each of these cases involved a comparable interorganizational structure in a comparable city pursuing the same goals through the same funding mechanism, it becomes clear that the nature of the environment itself is not determined or predicted by the missions of the organizations in question. Inevitably, there are cultural factors embedded in the histories of the organizations' relations, the politics of the city, and the practices of the communities involved. Tight control structures may function as a mechanism for reducing uncertainty in situations where the parties have not built a base of trust and goodwill, or, as in Atlanta, where some of the participants actually appeared to be trying to undermine others. As Dill explains,

> Because the technical requirements of medicine are high and place performance pressures on hospitals that affect decisions by patients and physicians to use them, hospitals can be said to operate in a stronger technical environment than do less technical social service and community-based care agencies, such as those leading the projects in Dallas and Atlanta. These may, then, have translated into the performance pressures expressed within the Miami project.
>
> Such an interpretation is at best incomplete, however, for it ignores some basic details. First, nothing in the operations of the Miami project is inherently more technical than in the other sites; . . . moreover, all three projects have had to find ways of dealing with the different norms and rationalities brought together by working with coalitions of health care, social service, and community-based organizations. (1994, 363–64)

Dill concludes that prior interorganizational experience in Dallas led to a shared cultural framework built around the "institutional myth" of consensus and coordination both within the nonprofit sector and between the nonprofits and the public health sector. Atlanta suffered from a lack of such a history and no shared framework, so everything had to be carefully negotiated or disputed, particularly across sector boundaries. Miami, the extreme other end, was hampered by a history of disjuncture between the well-funded hospital that became the lead agency—which did not need the grant money or otherwise need to compromise with the community groups—and the community groups, which did not function cohesively to begin with. The hospital had high institutional legitimacy and considerable resources. The community groups lacked the extrainstitutional resources necessary to make a dent in the hospital's practices or priorities.

There are many differences between the cases of community organizing in New York City and elsewhere during the same period. Included among them are the differences in political environments and cultural histories that Dill examined. The New York groups operated in an interorganizational environment characterized by a high degree of domain consensus (general agreement over functions and roles) and normative interaction. They had agencies of their own that could compete for legitimacy with the public health sector, as well as organizations whose main work often seemed to be attacking the legitimacy of state agents. Seemingly overwhelming all of these, however, even in New York, was the single factor of a competitive, formal funding program with relatively deep pockets. It may not be much of an exaggeration to say that before 1991, the question for community organizations was how to respond to HIV/AIDS, and afterward, it was how to respond to CARE Act requests for proposals.

The use of financial incentives to limit political organizing is not new or unique to large programs. Most of the community-based organizations participating in the consortia, or otherwise involved in getting and spending money, are incorporated as nonprofit corporations chartered in a given state. The usual designation for a tax-exempt charitable or social organization, under federal tax law, is 501(c)(3). As charitable organizations redistributing private money for the public good, these groups are not taxed on their "income." They are, however, confined to a narrow form of activity that excludes participating in politics. Should they cross the line from service organization to interest group, they could lose their tax status. This distinction has practical purposes. Charities can reasonably claim privileges that others, acting on their own behalf, cannot. But a direct and probably not unintended effect, as argued by Jeffrey Berry and David Arons (2003), is that in the world of political lobbying—political voice—only those groups most in need of an organized advocate are constrained in this way against having one. Businesses and individual property owners and investors organize to increase their political leverage, often through the paid services of lobbying firms. It is an investment that can yield higher profits. Nonprofit organizations representing people in need are expected not to do any of that. Each individual group must make a choice: whether to make the case for what needs to be done (act politically), or do it themselves (provide services). The two can coexist only at the interorganizational level. Consortia, therefore, can be extremely powerful and multivocal if the membership is reasonably diverse and they are not all bound to a single set of organizational goals and practices. A funded consortium without a lead agency or a joint mission statement could actually foster political voice while providing social services. The CARE Act consortia did not.

Carl Milofsky, among others, has described comparable phenomena occurring in other broad community mobilizations such as the War on Poverty relief and community empowerment efforts of the 1960s. In that case, federal support for the "maximum feasible participation" (Moynihan 1969) of community groups supported local interests, but at the same time, the institutionalization of a single, distant, and competitive funding stream yielded considerable reorganizing within the target communities. Primarily, groups that had been highly embedded in, and focused on, their local communities had to not only reorient themselves to the priorities of outside agencies but also to compete for grants against groups with whom they shared a considerable overlap of interests and values. Generally speaking,

> in an environment in which other organizations aggressively seek out and attempt to control available resources, passive organizations which are not independently wealthy are soon starved out. Rather than starve, many community organizations have taken on organizational characteristics which allow them to compete better in the mass social system. They narrow the activities they undertake in an effort to claim to be sole providers in some part of the service system. They expand those services for which it is easy to show efficient functioning in hopes of convincing distant resource providers that there are well run and accountable programs. (Milofsky 1988, 30)

The positive effect of both federal support and community reorganization is that local collective actors can successfully undertake large and important projects. Things can get done that were previously unimaginable. That is one of the reasons, not the only one, that the groups knowingly and deliberately choose to reorganize themselves. But the costs are also significant, for the groups, for the communities, and for the people who need the organizations.

> All of these changes often make small local nonprofits unsuited to community building because they no longer encourage and reward participation. Their decision making processes no longer are forums in which interpersonal disputes with origins outside the organization are worked out. They are no longer free to shift goals to meet immediate community needs. (Milofsky 1988, 30)

In short, they are no longer embedded in their communities. That, of course, is the underlying point made by informants in resource-poor HIV/AIDS groups who criticize the larger organizations for having expensive furniture or dress codes. Professionalizing—"going corporate"—is a way of stepping out of "the community." In cultural terms, it is disempowering.

The issue of empowerment and disempowerment was, of course, central to the case of federal support for Community Action Programs (CAPs) under the

War on Poverty. The attempt by the Office of Economic Opportunity to empower community action groups, without the participation of local power brokers and sometimes at their expense, might well have been the principal reason for the failure of so many of the CAPs (Greenstone and Peterson 1973). The unique aspect of that system, which has not been repeated since, was to provide funds directly to "indigenous" community groups in order to make them less accountable to local government and even allow them to build their own power blocs capable of challenging local elites. The more conventional system, represented by almost all federal grant systems since then, including the Ryan White CARE Act, has been to make funding dependent on the kind of formal grants-writing procedures in which government and the larger private institutions specialize, thereby compelling smaller groups to seek their collaboration. Far from being able to use federal money to bypass these institutions, the community action groups must convince the institutions that they can work within the system. They have to make themselves accountable to others in the bureaucracy and therefore less accountable to their communities of origin.

THE LIMITS OF COOPERATION

When the first community-based organizations sought to work with governmental agencies in the early days of HIV/AIDS, they were operating in a void. The groups expected that the health and social services domain would take the initiative and that the volunteers would ensure that implementation was handled correctly. They sought to educate the government about the needs of the community while educating the community about their own rights and responsibilities. In the familiar pattern of civil society mobilization, they identified an organizational space in between the state and the citizen defined around various social identity constructs.

Under the consortia system, community groups became responsible for implementation of the state's AIDS policies. Therefore, they were no longer in a position to protest implementation questions. Even an independent or activist arm of the community could not vigorously attack such problems as discrimination in the delivery of goods and services without risking that the state would simply punish the groups that were actually delivering the goods. Organizations that were formally connected had to speak with one voice. Those that were not linked remained isolated. Interorganizational relations became less dynamic and flexible.

Service contracts have a co-optive influence (Selznick 1949). CBOs that adopt an antagonistic posture while holding contracts risk not only losing those contracts, but they may also find their entire consortia threatened with dissolution. Organizations in such relationships can no longer even effectively challenge policy makers with statistics about the extent of unmet needs in the community, for it is they who are failing to meet those needs. An individual organization may choose not to participate, but it can be replaced. In the case of HIV/AIDS consortia, available funding engendered crowding in a field that was once sparse. This change introduced new resources to the field and more options for people living with HIV/AIDS, while divesting the most active community agencies of much of their status and influence.

More to the point, having successfully made its case that the state should take responsibility, the community lost its "moral monopoly" (Jasper 1997). In gaining tangible benefits, they lost an important part of their social power, which had come from the claim of having been abandoned. Subsequently, the organized community could only lobby for more money, which placed them in no special position on a very long line. As Douglas Crimp wrote, "How often do we hear the list recited: poverty, crime, drugs, homelessness, and AIDS? AIDS is no longer an emergency. It's merely a permanent disaster" (1992, 5).

WHERE ARE THEY NOW?

The community consortia model grew throughout the 1990s. Federal appropriations for the spectrum of CARE Act provisions rose from $220.5 million in 1991 to nearly $1.6 billion in 2000, with an increase from three major programs (Titles I through III) to six (HRSA 2002). Throughout this period of increased federal participation, the model remained centered on the role of CBOs, with significant input from the organized community into HIV policies. By 1999, the New York City Department of Health maintained "more than 200 contracts with over 130 community-based organizations, hospitals, clinics and other HIV/AIDS service providers" (New York City Department of Health 1999). Indeed, the acceptance of community activists and advocates in the formal policy process after 1990 was so unquestioned that by the early 1990s, major media sources were referring to it as a "monopoly," decrying the "excessive" influence of the powerful gay lobby in HIV/AIDS, seemingly at the expense of heterosexual women, people of color, and especially children (Booth 2000).

The initial AHSP (demonstration project) funding was intended for start-up costs rather than for long-term funding. Outside of New York, most of the surviving consortia shifted from AHSP support to state funding through HRSA in the early 1990s, with development plans appropriate for the requirements of the CARE Act (Allen et al. 1995). Forty states established Ryan White Title I or Title II consortia within the first grant year. All of the AHSP sites still functioning in 1994 were receiving federal funds to continue (Mor et al. 1994, 145). By 1995, CARE Act funding had become the largest source of revenue for HIV/AIDS service providers in New York. At least half of the extant New York City CBOs examined for this study received Title I funding as part of their participation in service consortia within the first few years of the program (Bureau of Ryan White CARE Services 1995). The AHSP sites served as the basis on which the CARE Act consortia were developed. The network of organized community groups in the city formed the material out of which the consortia were constructed.

The availability of CARE Act funding had a substantial impact on interorganizational relations in the HIV/AIDS field in New York, without completely removing the community's sense of initiative. At the Community Health Project (CHP), for example, they distinguished between the CBOs that they worked with and those with whom they had linkages. "To their credit," they explained, funders "want to see who you're connected to in the community as validation for your program." In response, CHP signed contracts with CBOs that needed care provision connections as a form of endorsement. "Even if they don't use it, it's there by agreement. Other organizations have nothing on paper, but we talk to them all the time." (Since the time of this interview, the Community Health Project reorganized as a much larger and more formally operated multiservice agency known as the Callen-Lorde Community Health Services Center, whose $3 million budget mostly comes from government grants.)[2] At Housing Works, a nominally activist group with a considerable number of service programs, the CARE Act was far too long in coming. Many of the ancillary services that Housing Works had developed came about in order to fill the gaps that they expected the city to cover. The group had also sought a kind of consortium model. They had initially assumed that once their clients were housed, "we could link with other agencies" for drug treatment and medical advocacy. At that time, however, the non-HIV organizations were not interested in working with them. Once those links came into being, through government intervention, Housing Works began to rely on them, though much more of their income derives from private contributions and billable program services.

Both of these groups contained significant service delivery functions and had therefore been seeking a stable source of government or other funding. The already-existing activist activities at Housing Works were not significantly affected, since the group had already found its own balance of services and politics. Similarly, CHP, with its emphasis on medical care services, easily and readily took advantage of the restructuring of the community network to establish additional linkages, which had already been a primary goal of the group.

Like Housing Works, the People with AIDS Coalition of New York (PWAC/NY) had also been operating on many fronts with different survival strategies. The strategies were not always completely effective; the group underwent several major reorganizations since its founding and has since merged itself out of existence. The original PWAC was a leader in the empowerment movement and mostly provided support groups and "safe spaces" for group members. (The organization was made up of people living with HIV/AIDS, so they did not have clients.) When the organizers decided to expand into new directions, they launched a separate organization called Body Positive (BP). BP overlapped in function with PWAC, but the primary mission of BP was to publish the magazine *Body Positive*. This publication targeted a different readership than that of the popular *People with AIDS Coalition Newsline*. PWAC/NY pursued many goals but effectively compartmentalized them. In the final year of independent operation, they received government grants for slightly over half of their approximately $1 million annual budget.

Body Positive also expanded into multiple areas and communities, partnering with other groups for education and support services. In 2000, BP and PWAC/NY merged, with the Body Positive organization taking on PWAC's mission and programs. The 2001 annual budget for the organization in this form was almost $1.3 million, with nearly $840,000 coming from the state and federal government sources.

The Minority Task Force on AIDS (MTFA) always had an advocacy function but has concentrated much more heavily on expanding service availability to more marginal communities of need. Originally a kind of umbrella group seeking to connect people with existing service organizations, expand the horizons of those existing groups, and support the growth of additional services most needed by communities of color in the wake of HIV/AIDS, MTFA currently provides a wide array of housing and education services within and well outside of New York City. Supported almost entirely by government grants, MTFA spends between $4.5 and $5 million per year on housing services, legal advocacy, education, and family services.

Recent data on the organizations' income sources were not readily available for all of the study groups discussed here, but of the ones with public tax records, most have grown significantly.[3] In those cases, state funding, including both federal CARE Act support and state grants made through the AIDS Institute, constitute large but not always dominant sources of support. Among the groups most dependent on government support were the HIV Law Project, which received $800,000 in grants out of a total 2002–2003 budget of $1.2 million, and the Hispanic AIDS Forum, with $3.2 million out of an approximate budget of

$3.5 million (2001–2002) based on grants. Approximately 90 percent of Positive Health Project's $1 million budget also came from grants during that period, as did the majority of revenues for the service organizations Momentum Project and the Foundation for Research on Sexually Transmitted Diseases (FROST'D).

More commonly, government grants provide one leg of the groups' incomes, particularly for those providing billable services. God's Love We Deliver received $2.7 million of their $8.35 million annual budget, CHP took in $2.3 million out of about $7 million, and Housing Works received $1.8 million in grants while taking in almost $9 million from all other sources. Gay Men's Health Crisis (GMHC), with its remarkable $21.2 million in total revenue in 2001–2002, received $7.8 million in government support, which is just over one-third of all income. Several of the organizations exist to raise and redistribute money and so have no service-related grants, while alternative therapy groups like Direct AIDS Alternative Information Resource (DAAIR) do not undertake the kinds of services for which grant money is available.

With over 121,000 cases of AIDS reported in New York City by December 2004, and 20,000 more living with confirmed HIV diagnoses (Bureau of AIDS Epidemiology 2005), the service organizations in the field have had to become multimillion-dollar corporations. To do so has required them to participate as fully as possible in the world of grantsmanship—applying for large government grants, altering services according to what is both supported and needed, and providing accountability to funders and regulators. While those few organizations that work on conceptual political and social issues can remain apart from such changes in the field, and purely political groups have no choice but to remain outside of it, service-oriented groups do not have that choice. On their own, even with a generous community of private supporters, they cannot fulfill what has become a public function. The once private, local, and sometimes informally run nonprofits that began in someone's living room or a church basement have become institutionalized on the front lines of a massive service system. The question was not whether HIV/AIDS care would be institutionalized, but rather who would be doing the work when it happened.

CONCLUSION

CARE Act consortia brought together the state, the public health sector, and the affected communities in a new partnership based on the goal of helping people living with HIV/AIDS. This is, in fact, an important part of what the activist and advocacy CBOs had asked for. Certain aspects of the new state-community partnership were imposed on the CBOs. In other respects, however, it was merely the next, more complex stage in the ongoing negotiation of relations and responsibilities.

The self-generated network of community-based action gave the CBOs multiple points of contact with the state, multiple sites of action, and hundreds of redundant, interleaving connections through which actions could be coordinated without central control. Why, then, did the organizations in the various consortia studies consistently move away from a community-based model of organization? Three factors must be considered in order to answer this question. First, most of the consortia had been established in cities that lacked the kind of indigenous infrastructure that occurred on such a large scale in New York. The most affected communities, for whatever combination of reasons, could not put together a self-sustained structure of support for all those in need. Therefore, they needed to join in a larger structure. Second, even in New York City, where community mobilization was at its peak, needs were also greatest. The community response took more than ten years to grow with no appreciable outside source of monetary support, reliant on volunteers, many of whom had since died. Inevitably, the community needed to form linkages with outside agencies. However rapidly the community network had grown and however remarkable its accomplishments, its resource base was limited. It could not sustain the burden.

The third issue is simply that community organizations, regardless of internal support and internal pressures, do respond to external influences. As agencies of the institutional environment provide incentives for selective organizational forms, CBOs reorient themselves accordingly (DiMaggio and Powell 1991; Morgen 1986). As many groups all seek support from a single funding stream, competition does arise according to the terms set by the external agencies, mandated cooperation notwithstanding (Minkoff 1994).

An additional conclusion is more speculative but worth consideration. The availability of outside funds provided an incentive for non-HIV/AIDS CBOs, or non–community-based nonprofit agencies, to become involved in AIDS care. In Dallas, for example, "Ryan White set off a feeding frenzy" among service organizations that had previously avoided contact with HIV/AIDS (Bielefeld and Scotch 1996, 48). Indeed, that may be one of its accomplishments. As more groups entered into the HIV/AIDS care system, and as more social actors who did not share the histories and culture of the initiators entered the picture, it should not be surprising to find the field moving overall away from a community-centered approach.

The San Francisco model embraced a social service framework of organization among nonprofit organizations. Yet it provided room for some forms of community representation, particularly in the context of needs assessment. Many of the channels of communication and influence that the gay community in San Francisco maintained with the city and the Department of Health actually predated HIV/AIDS. For the largest organized community, then, the HIV/AIDS care partnership did not require significant additional attention to political voice. There were, of course, conflicts over who had voice or not, and at what cost. But there was a history of effective negotiation between the city and community-based organizations.

The post-Stonewall relations between the gay communities in New York and the city were more tense and sometimes openly hostile. Conditions were far worse for encounters between the city and drug users, particularly after the crack hysteria of the mid-1980s (which corresponded extremely closely to the height of AIDS hysteria). The community organizers were constrained by the city's distrust, or disdain, toward them and were empowered by their distrust, or disdain, for the city.

The New York urban action network did not quite generate an oppositional framework, although it depended on the presence of activists within the system. Among other functions, the activists helped to protect the field from the pressures of what Wolfgang Seibel (1989) called "mellow weakness"—the bind that states can place on nonprofit organizations by transferring responsibility to them for community problems that are beyond solution. The consortium model, by comparison, created exactly that dilemma. It strengthened the state-community partnership in the provision of services through a system that abjures political advocacy or activism. When its limitations were revealed, there wasn't much anyone in a community-based care network could do about it.

In the unique context of HIV/AIDS, in which community groups have created the only viable field of work, the state could not define its own role other than in contrast to the community. The New York community network had maintained a "safe" distance from state influence by keeping its antagonistic side active. This posture freed the state of the obligation to work with the community. In contrast to the consortium model, in which the state reduced its own perceived responsibility by offloading the burden onto CBOs, the cooperative-antagonistic (or insider-outsider) relationship that the New York community established with the state allowed the state to refuse responsibility altogether. But once a government program was implemented, there was little or no choice for any of the agencies involved. If the state had offered the community a form of partnership and the community had refused, then the community would risk permanently taking on full responsibility for HIV/AIDS care without state aid. Having spent years defining and demonstrating the need for government action in response to HIV/AIDS, the urban action network was at last undone by the government's acquiescence. Through initiatives like the Ryan White CARE Act, the state made the community an offer they couldn't refuse.

NOTES

1. The 501(c)(3) designation is given to certain "charitable organizations" in order to confer tax-exempt status. Exemptions may be granted to nonprofit organizations serving the public good in any of several defined ways, and these organizations are mostly restricted from engaging in political activities.

2. These and other budget figures come tax records, form 1990, submitted by the organizations in question between 2000 and 2003.

3. The IRS form 990, the "Return of Organization Exempt from Income Tax" statement, is not required for groups that either pay income tax or whose gross income is under $25,000.

Part Three

NETWORKS AND
CONTENTIOUS POLITICS

Chapter Seven

Urban Action Networks

In chapter 1, I presented evidence that people living with HIV/AIDS were at greater risk due to the state's failure to establish a national agenda in response to HIV/AIDS. In chapter 6, I argued that something was lost when the state became actively involved in setting this agenda, not only within New York City but also in the larger AIDS policy domain. I do not intend to imply that the prospects or daily situations of people with HIV/AIDS were preferable when the organized community was left to its own resources. As one informant stated, "Epidemics happen at the community level. Prevention is not done on a community level." What I would like to suggest is that the organized community had derived a model of interorganizational relations that gave them surprising amounts of influence in the cultural politics of their particular policy domain. The later compromise in state-community relations acceded to many of the community's priorities in a form that reduced that influence. In order to understand how influence was reduced under the new configuration of relations, it is necessary to examine the conditions on which the old influence depended.

I introduced the term "urban action network" to define the relational processes that characterized the workings of the organized HIV/AIDS community. I use this term as an ideal type of an informally constituted interorganizational network capable of growth, coordination, and political action without a centralized control structure. This form of linkage allows and encourages multivocality and the simultaneous pursuit of multiple campaigns, to the mutual benefit of the participants as a collective. Urban action networks engage multiple organizations and constituencies in semicoordinated action within a single policy domain.

None of the elements of this network form are entirely new to this case study. Similar processes have been observed in women's activism, civil rights activism, and the environmental movement, for example (Buechler 1990; Freeman 1975; Haines 1984; Lichterman 1995; Morris 1984, 2000; Tarrow 1994). What is new is a combination of conditions that allowed this particular network to develop farther and faster than most, thereby revealing tendencies that had been present in many prior mobilizations but not as fully realized. Those enabling conditions may be termed scope, novelty, and slack.

Scope, in this context, refers to the diversity of the affected populations, and hence, the breadth and diversity of the "mobilization potential" (Klandermans 1993). The mobilization and growth of a network of community organizations requires a broad constituency on which to draw. The more narrowly a policy arena is defined, the more tightly the boundaries between those affected and everyone else are drawn. Leaders of nascent social movements have incentives to broaden their constituency and potential sources of allies by defining their issue as everyone's problem (Bearman and Everett 1993). Their opponents may seek to diminish the scope of a set of claims by characterizing the movement as a "special interest" issue. Of course, a mobilization cannot encompass everyone, or there would be no one to mobilize against. But organizers often claim to represent not just their communities but the public good.

The universality of the health emergency helped HIV/AIDS organizers to involve an extensive constituency of concerned citizens. Initial mobilization efforts were limited by the public perception of HIV/AIDS as a problem of "deviants," by the mass media's relative lack of coverage, and by the federal government's unwillingness to treat AIDS as a public problem. As we have seen, a considerable amount of early work by community actors was dedicated to "normalizing AIDS" and to establishing a more general language for a public discussion. These efforts were followed by extensive efforts at community building and community expansion. Several factors in conjunction helped to overcome the marginalization of HIV/AIDS in the public eye. Among them were the active involvement of media friendly organizations such as Mothers' Voices and the aggressive public relations campaigns of groups as diverse as the AIDS Coalition to Unleash Power (ACT UP) and Gay Men's Health Crisis (GMHC). Outside of the community network, the visible support of celebrity spokespersons and the increasing investment in medical research nationwide also broadened the scope of AIDS awareness.

Novelty provides collective actors with flexibility. When an issue is new, innovation is encouraged and even required. Interorganizational networking within a policy domain can be more dynamic if there is no preexisting field of work defined around the issue or subsuming the issue. The organizational forms that individual community groups may take on do not have to be at all unique for the interorganizational processes to be new. Organizers mobilize supporters around shared meanings within familiar repertoires of action (Tilly

1996). Flexibility derives from the fact that a set of relations, organizational forms, and domain practices has not yet been institutionalized. Once a set of practices, forms, and relations has been fixed—once work in a field has acquired its own normative ways of doing things—it may become disruptive to go against these norms (DiMaggio and Powell 1983).

HIV/AIDS organizers adopted familiar forms for most of the individual community initiatives they pursued while creating a constantly shifting field of work. Until their missions were fixed by service consortia contracts, organizers in the HIV/AIDS field were free to redefine and reinvent themselves each time the political, social, or medical context shifted. Activism, service, and advocacy were all familiar forms of work for community groups, but the development of treatment activism as a form of advocacy, or buyers' clubs as part of an empowerment process, were powerful innovations that shook up the field of work. The diversity of efforts by organizations participating in debates on syringe exchange outmaneuvered their opponents, even during the height of the war on drugs. The combination of insider and outsider techniques made allies of the community's enemies without diminishing the virtual power of the protest actions.

Slack implies that the organizational identity of a field and the identity of the roles within it develop indigenously, without significant organized opposition. A nascent movement without an organized opposition has the freedom to define its issues in its own terms and according to the experiences of its members. This phenomenon had been observed among the consciousness-raising groups of the women's movement in the 1970s, who found their voice in small meetings defined by and for women where one's personal experiences were primary, where one had "free space" to speak without criticism or questions (Shreve 1989). Many social movements begin this way. In contrast, Black southerners had to hide and fight in order to protect the free spaces in which to cultivate a civil rights narrative in the early years of that movement (Couto 1993). But the period of free discourse may be limited. The often rapid establishment of a countermovement compels community organizations to harden their positions and limit their actions (Mansbridge 1986; Meyer and Staggenborg 1998).

The earliest organizations in the HIV/AIDS field defined a broad range of needs from research to service provision. They also defined spaces in the field in which it was not yet clear that action would be necessary. With the continued lack of a forceful government presence, the organized community expanded to fill all of these spaces. In many cases, individuals participated in organized action in several different locations within the field simultaneously. This freedom lasted almost to the moment when the Ryan White Comprehensive AIDS Resources Emergency funding began to flow.

DYNAMIC NETWORK PROCESSES

The urban action network model is a loose, nonfederated structure in which the internal boundaries between the component parts are fluid, participants do not have to choose to align themselves with only one set of forms or goals, and individual organizations can contribute to work in many areas. A community that is so organized may pursue multiple claims and multiple forms of relations with different government agencies within a single policy arena. In theory, the same flexibility and multivocality would be available in any institutional domain, political or otherwise. Any external or internal factors that compel organizations in the network to formalize their connections or to exaggerate the differences between them would also function to impede the informal links out of which the dynamic system of relations is composed. Once "fixed" in this way, the relational system will be transformed into a "solid" structure. It is, therefore, the dynamicism of the informal system of relations that makes it unique.

The advent of HIV/AIDS in New York City mobilized a broad constituency of affected peoples, some of whom had access to significant resources. Left to their own devices for a surprisingly long time, these organizers were able to mobilize a wide net of groups into a functioning interorganizational network. The functioning of the network as a network required an active web of connections running throughout the field of work. It required that as the community grew larger and more diverse, the participants would remain connected or would form connections. The mechanisms by which this occurred had little to do with HIV/AIDS. The crucial means by which the community defined and manipulated a shared space—encountered here as *splitting*, *outreach*, and *enrollment*—were dynamic interorganizational processes that may be found in almost any growing network. The community of organizations worked as a unit, a single field of action, not simply because of shared interest but because it was networked.

A network can grow as a result of *splitting*, the division of a member organization into two or more groups. The simplest example would be that of a small splinter group leaving its parent organization, in which case the original name, most of the functions, and most of the organizational links of the original organization would remain attached to the parent organization while the new group emerged with a limited subset of the original mission and resources. At the very least, the new organization would be tied to the network through the single link to its parent, even though the relationship might be somewhat strained. As a worst-case scenario, one could imagine a case where the split followed a complete organizational breakdown such that the two groups would end up in a state of outright hostility, with no shared members, no supportive interactions at all on issues of common concern, and no common links to other community-based organizations (CBOs). In such a scenario, the split would serve to reduce rather than expand the network. But even in this case it would be reasonable for some of the interorganizational links to transfer with the subset of the organization to the new location, akin to the process by which a couple undergoing a hostile divorce divide their mutual friends into exclusive groups. Although antagonistic, the two emergent organizational entities would then both maintain ties to the existing network. The worst-case scenario would entail two groups each claiming to "really" embody the original group, with each denying the validity of the other.

In any less extreme case of an organizational split, some subset of personnel would remain with each group, likely including a degree of overlap. Specific elements of the ongoing mission of the initial organization would transfer to the new offshoot and would thus be demoted in the priorities of the old, again reasonably including an overlap of interests. Through the fact of these two overlaps, some number of organizational ties would transfer to the emergent organization, but not necessarily at the cost of the original links. Barring extreme conditions the initial organization would be replaced by two tightly bound organizations occupying different niches within the same subfield. In network terms, the new corporate entities would remain in the same cluster as the single entity they have replaced, with redundant ties to the rest of the cluster, thereby increasing the size of the cluster without necessarily reducing its density. In practical terms, two independent groups would exist where previously there had been one.

Splitting may also be viewed as a mechanism for loosening the bonds between the parent organization and its field of work, thereby increasing both the diversity and the flexibility of the network. "'Ties' tie you down," as Jane Mansbridge (1993, 374) observed. Launching a new organizational effort clears away some degree of acquired routine or obligation attendant to the initial group's network location and history and may help to create distance between the new group and the expectations of the old. Splits also serve to help an organization break out of a course of action with which it has become identified but which later becomes a constraint. Within the organization of women's activism in the 1970s, for example, Roberta Spalter-Roth and Ronnee Schreiber found that the boundary between "insider" and "outsider" tactics had become institutionalized, to the detriment of the movement. "Once the tactical choice had been made to use a professional insider style, however, controversy arose when specific organizations tried to return to confrontational outsider techniques" (Spalter-Roth and Schreiber 1995, 114). An organization that was associated with a single political posture could not easily, under the rubric of that organizational identity, reverse itself. The emergence of new organizations out of the base of the existing ones, however, allows collective actors to alter their strategies without undermining their existing work.

Splitting loosens bonds, but it need not sever them. The relationship between the originating and the emergent organizations may be characterized as a parent-child relationship in which the parent organization might well have an interest in helping the fledgling group to grow. It would be surprising if an organization, having given rise to a particular effort out of which the new group is born, lost interest in the effort altogether. This remains valid even as we expect the new organization to take a strong position on the common issues, differentiating itself from its parent (Tarrow 1994, 20). The implied support relations between the two can also be viewed as a resource to the community of organizations. "The problem for a new organization," Wim Wiewel and Albert Hunter have observed, "is that it has nothing to offer but promises. But if it is grafted onto or buds from an existing organization, it can trade on the credit of the older organization and thus accumulate the resources that will allow it to reciprocate" (1985, 486). The interest that the parent organization demonstrates in the new group can be as important to the establishment of the emergent effort as the interpersonal ties that the founders transfer with them.

The second network growth process is *outreach*, which is analogous to the recruitment of new individuals into an existing organization. In the case of community-based networks, existing organizations may identify a need and then seek out new agencies to help them address it. Service organizations expanding into a new location, for example, can make contact with service organizations already working in that location, establishing a channel through which the local groups could later collaborate with the existing network (Spencer 1993). The least active form of outreach occurs when a networked organization publishes a request for proposal (RFP) in order to support the work of outside agencies through a controlled point of entry and attached to a limited function. Even this limited case serves to bridge gaps between the network and areas of work outside the network, creating a small, immediate expansion and opening new opportunities for future growth. The more general form of the process occurs when a subset of networked organizations invite the participation of others in a new or expanding effort, leaving room for the new groups to establish their own place in the larger structure.

In the event of outreach, the new organization may itself be embedded within a different network of its own. The new link, therefore, would create a bridge to span the two networks, providing a point of contact among all of the participants of the new network and any point in the original. The connection would provide a new path for the flow of information and other resources between two sets of organizations where an infrastructure has already been defined. The organizations that create the bridge, spanning what Ronald Burt

(1992) has defined as a "structural hole," inherently become more central in the new, larger network than either was likely to have been in the separate ones. Thus, organizations may benefit in both the short and long term by establishing interorganizational relations.

Outreach, however, could be perceived by some as a form of colonization in which the larger network, seeking diversity, offers marginal groups the opportunity to reorient themselves to what might be considered the mainstream or power base of the active community (Spalter-Roth and Schreiber 1995, 122). The network would expand, with possible opportunities for boundary-spanning activities and mixing of individuals across constituency groups, but the immediate effect would be to introduce new sources of interorganizational conflict. Successful outreach across a broad constituency can expand the power, resources, and flexibility of a network of organizations; less successful outreach can be a destructive force.

Outreach may gather groups one at a time, or it may be organized as an attempt to wrap many small efforts into a single wide net or federation. The latter is a common strategy among community mobilizations, often described as building bridges, community outreach, strategic partnerships, or coalition building. Prominent examples include the 1966 formation of the National Organization for Women (NOW) as an umbrella group linking hundreds of local organizations, and the 1960 organization of the Student Nonviolent Coordinating Committee (SNCC) as a network among campus peace groups. Such structural hubs or umbrella organizations are often designed to be quasi-permanent points of exchange among related groups in a single policy domain, and they imply an increase in hierarchy. Temporary, event-centered coalitions are also popular mechanisms by which a community of organizations may expand with less hierarchy. Coalitions bring diverse groups into contact around an issue of concern to each of them, with the assumption that a shared pool of resources and a greater assortment of perspectives can accomplish something that the separate agencies on their own could not. Interorganizational outreach efforts create connections that may endure after the structures in which they were formed, the coalitions, have formally disbanded. What matters here is that the organizations share enough of a collective identity or intent to form a coalition, not that the coalition should become permanent.

The third network growth mechanism may be called *enrollment*, which is the counterpart to recruitment. Enrollment occurs when independent CBOs or local groups seek contact with networked organizations in order to expand their own venues or resource bases. The emerging organizational effort, the group's branching out into a new area, may tap into the organizational base of the network in a manner that is compatible with existing efforts in order to construct its new identity or role. A geographically local organization may seek contact with a national network of related groups, as in the case of a women's advocacy group seeking to join NOW. A relatively small group organized around a particular issue of interest to its community might enroll the support of an existing network from within the community. An organization concerned with discrimination against gay employees within a particular industry, for example, might wish to join forces with the Gay and Lesbian Alliance against Defamation (GLAAD) and its network of supporters. Additionally, an organization or network engaged in one form of work, such as service provision, may seek an alliance with an existing network of organizations of a different form, such as advocacy, where both sets of organizations serve the interests of a single constituency. Although many studies of social movements have situated their focal movement organizations within a multi-organizational field of supportive nonmovement organizations (Aminzade 1995; Gould 1991; McAdam 1988; Rosenthal et al. 1990), few studies have examined the processes through which those linkages were formed (but see Diani 2001; Philips 1991). Enrollment is one such process.

Outreach and enrollment occur after a network of community groups has already been mobilized within a recognized domain. They link organizational actors across movement or sector boundaries. From the perspective of new network members, the preexisting organizational base for the expanded mobilization is easily identified. The network can be located. Similar processes, wherein individuals attached to one social movement organization follow organizational links to become supporters of a different movement, have been described as "social movement spillover" (Meyer and Whittier 1994), or as the expansion of "social movement sectors" (Buechler 1990). Work in the newer domain may even reactivate links and resource pools developed in the older domain. The remaining interorganizational relations among relatively quiescent movement organizations, following a major defeat, for example, have been shown to provide the organizational base out of which renewed activism may later grow (Taylor 1989). Even terrorist groups have been traced to incubation periods within "a wider social movement sector" (Della Porta 1988, 156).

Over time, as the member organizations continue to function as independent groups, a network also functions as a network. We commonly speak of the use of existing links to form new contacts as "networking." The existence of a network structure creates opportunities for individual members (nodes) that are not directly connected to form such links. This process may be called "network consolidation," with reference to the ability of the network to generate new internal ties and to function as a single entity with common interests. Interorganizational networking functions include the exchange of personnel and information; participation in joint ventures; redistribution of one another's literature; normalized relationships of client, member, or customer referrals (whichever is appropriate); and cross listings or postings of one another's events. Linked organizations experience more opportunities for contact, heightened awareness of the work that each performs, and the ability to draw upon one another as resources. Unlike rival organizations or business competitors, coparticipants in a policy-minded network have incentives to share at least some resources with an eye to the larger interests.

A field of work can grow or shrink. New organizations can be established; old ones may fail. As new efforts are organized, the field of work becomes more complex. This complexity does not only entail an increase in the amount of work that occurs within the network space or the number of people doing the work. Each new set of goals and forms of action alters the definition of the field of work itself, thus altering the nature of the network. When new efforts emerge from recombinations of existing groups within the field, the resources of the network may be spread more thinly. As new ties are formed from within the existing network to other groups with related interests, resources may be brought in. Such resources may include expertise, materials, or simply fresh blood and fresh ideas.

Organization as Launchpad

Treatment Action Group's (TAG's) departure from ACT UP "left the organization poorer" (*New Yorker* 1992). But it was neither unprecedented nor antithetical to the workings of ACT UP. The "iron law of oligarchy" (Michels 1968) notwithstanding, ACT UP/NY did not pursue its own viability or seek to institutionalize its own role—quite the opposite. ACT UP consistently risked its own existence in order to disrupt the institutional links that bound other social actors into a fixed location within the state-community system of relations. The activists affiliated under the ACT UP designation were encouraged to use the group as a launching point for action on any issue that they felt was necessary. If their efforts took root, the offshoots took on independent lives. This unique organizational form, which relied on their position as an activist hub within a broader field, actively fostered organizational splits as a strategy for network growth.

As the working group on housing shifted their attention from activism to service and advocacy, for example, they too moved away from their ACT UP form. Having acquired a new constituency and requiring budgets that ACT UP could not support, they separated to form Housing Works. Housing Works maintained a strong connection to its activist roots while putting much of its attention to the world of federal and city funding. They received considerable amounts of housing assistance for homeless people with HIV/AIDS, a population that had previously been more likely to be evicted from public housing than offered emergency space. The Needle Exchange committee gave rise to five syringe exchange programs throughout the city, each of which incorporated as an independent group. Through their nearly ubiquitous presence at every forum, conference, and media event during their first five years, ACT UP/NY further fostered the growth of the organized community in less direct ways.

Stand Up Harlem, now defunct, also began as a spin-off from ACT UP. Yet that may not speak as well of the interrelations across cultural boundaries as other links do. When founder Louis Jones left ACT UP, it was reportedly a response to "the difficulties in trying to find a place for people of color in ACT UP."[1]

For Mothers' Voices, ACT UP provided inspiration, technical advice, and a point of contrast. Mothers' Voices began in 1991 with five mothers of people with AIDS talking in a kitchen on Long Island. The mothers had all been in attendance at a New York University presentation on promising developments in AIDS prophylaxis when ACT UP had tried to take over the proceedings. Initially disturbed by the activists' disruptive chants (they shouted "I don't have two years" at a researcher discussing the drug research process), the women "realized that the activists were right." Their children were likely to die before the treatments under development became available.

The organizers of Mothers' Voices also realized that most of the people in the room and elsewhere weren't listening to ACT UP and that someone had to "put a personal face on AIDS" that could appeal to the mainstream. They cultivated their best PTA image, not to distance themselves from activism but to add a new dimension to it. "We've said to ACT UP, 'we're just you in sheep's clothing. We can open doors that you can't.'" A GMHC staff member described Mothers' Voices and Housing Works as "both radical and conservative. Mothers' Voices are really radical in purpose, conservative in appearance. . . . Housing Works is more like the other way around."

Mothers' Voices recognized that parents of people living with HIV/AIDS and of those who have died are often as angry and willing to commit to action as are the younger activists. Unlike the street activists, however, the mothers could get appointments with their congressional representatives and make presentations at school and church groups. "We are the advocates to change public policy," one of the founders asserted. Beginning with the premise that letter writing "turns people into activists," Mothers' Voices initiated the Mothers' Day Card, signed by families of those affected by HIV and mailed to the White House each year with a plea for governmental action. Each new card campaign mobilized new parents interested in political action against HIV/AIDS. Mothers' Voices increased the level of activism by seemingly bypassing the AIDS community altogether.

LOCATIONS OF DISPLACED ACTION

Observing the growth and development of a new field of nonprofit organizing such as the HIV/AIDS organizations examined in this study, one can identify a trajectory wherein an organization's location reflects both its goals and its relations to the larger field. GMHC, ACT UP/NY, and TAG, for example, pursued different types of missions within a shared community, even as each enacted a different understanding of whom that community included. Between them, they provided organizational centers for service provision, activism, and advocacy, respectively, each of which relates to a different approach to the state. Each form of relationship—service provider, activist, and advocate—provides insight into the multifaceted dynamics associated with the link between the state and the organized community.

Service organizations like GMHC experienced the benefits and constraints inherent in cooperative "insider" relations with state agencies. GMHC sponsored conferences and community forums that brought state funders and service agencies into direct contact with street-level community service providers. Leaders of community-based AIDS service organizations in New York have served on the advisory boards of city agencies, thereby acquiring routine access to local and state policy processes. Their "closeness" to city and state institutions led some to question whether they had disembedded themselves from their community of origin even as it solidified the group's ability to represent "the community" to government.

The activists in ACT UP/NY and other political groups experienced firsthand the opportunities and constraints that come from outsider locations. They neither advised the city nor sought its support. Instead, through their rallies, newsletters, e-mail alerts, and phone activation networks, they channeled the virtual power of the affected communities into media events and civil disobedience in an ongoing effort to keep the government "honest." Operating in public, without offices or staff, facing arrest and violence, the group placed itself "on the street" and away from the boardrooms.

Advocacy organizations in policy domains, such as TAG, had the opportunity to occupy a mediating location. Within research and policy arenas, they could speak legitimately as community representatives without actually organizing a constituency or tarnishing their personal connections through protests or threats. Concurrently, their middle position made the treatment activists valuable allies to the public health sector. Within community forums, they explained medical options and standards of care to rooms full of people living with HIV/AIDS, using their own blood assays as visual aids, partially overcoming the taint of the health sector's history of neglect or outright hostility toward the affected communities. They straddled the territory between the public and private sectors.

The characteristics of the groups in this case study suggest the forms of organization in the different strata of any such action network. Thus GMHC exemplifies the subfield of service organizations that have grown around it and most closely defines the type. ACT UP/NY was the leading activist organization with connections to other less prominent groups of similar form. It adopted the familiar form of a grassroots protest organization while choosing an implementation particular to the needs of its members. TAG coordinated its work with a handful of other New York City nonprofit organizations (NPOs) where the groups' missions overlap. However, only TAG worked exclusively within a mediating model.

HIV/AIDS-related NPOs collectively defined a variety of locations with regard to the state before formalizing a single system of relations. The sequence of forms of work adopted by the nonprofit community groups revealed the negotiable status of state-community systems. This negotiation process indicates that discrete organizational strategies depend on both the structure of organizational fields at the collective level and the configuration of relations between fields and their environments. Their interdependencies demonstrate why private organizations in a policy domain sought to work both with and against the state and how they were able to do both.

The history of HIV/AIDS-related community-based NPOs offers further insights for scholars of nonprofit organizations. The ambivalence of the state's response for the first ten years or so of HIV/AIDS in the United States was itself remarkable (Cuthbert 1990; Shilts 1987). The absence of a formal policy on an epidemic of such proportion left private organizations to define the public response to HIV/AIDS. Hence, the organizations in this field were able, or compelled, to form a complex set of interdependencies among themselves almost devoid of either interference or assistance from the public health sector. The configuration of nonprofit organizations was thus uniquely determined by community organizing for some years prior to becoming fixed in a set of institutionally defined relations with state agencies.

One could argue that the task of maintaining control over a diverse and growing population of interest groups would be untenable, and that fragmentation is inevitable. Such an argument would view diversity as a failure to organize. Instead, I view the formation of many forms of interorganizational relations as a strategic contribution by multiple organizations to a shared set of goals. The debates preceding the formation of both ACT UP/NY and TAG provide explicit examples. In both cases, organizers wished to expand their work into new areas using different tactics, but they feared that the new approach would compromise the benefits of their ongoing work. In both cases, community organizers pursued both strategies by expanding the field of organizations. The splits did not make everyone happy, but they served the collective interests of the organized community.

This multiorganizational process provides some degree of protection to community autonomy while allowing them to form necessary alignments with state agencies. By providing alternative forms within the same field, NPOs can represent their communities of origin, often against the interests of the state, without fostering an entirely hostile pattern of interaction. The state, which shares these interests in goods and services provided by the community-based service organizations, has incentives to encourage the growth of the independent third sector but not its independence (Deakin 1995). By funding nonprofits as its agent, the state gains a measure of control, thereby bringing the NPOs into the public system without taking responsibility for the success or failure of the organizations or their missions (Seibel 1989). Formal support relations therefore reduce the nonprofits' autonomy, but only for those organizations that participate in such relations.

Contemporary community organizers and sociologists share an awareness of the dangers inherent in working with state agencies. Co-optation is part of the language of mobilization, and NPOs must consistently renegotiate their relations with the state at each step of their development. For any given organization, the decision to position the group as either outsiders or insiders may be the most significant point in their life cycle. Yet, as many informants observed, "both are needed." Organizers in this study and elsewhere have come to recognize the strategic advantages inherent in multiple points of work with only loose ties between them (Edwards 1994).

Studies of professionalization in social movements, drawing on the resource mobilization tradition, have compared cooperative "insider" NPOs with outsider antagonists in order to ask which has more successfully mobilized their resources (Zald and McCarthy 1987). Not surprisingly, organizations that maintain routine contact with economic and political elites have more successfully attracted reliable sources of support. But such studies play down the significance of context (Hathaway and Meyer 1994). Mainstream and radical organizations are able to specialize in this way because each may relegate necessary functions to the other (Stoller 1997). In certain cases, which Herbert Haines called "the radical flank effect," increases in elite contributions to mainstream exchange partners have been directly attributed to recent activism by radical groups (Haines 1984; Jenkins and Eckert 1986; McAdam 1982). Where such a division of labor occurs, mediating organizations may attempt to manipulate the dichotomy to further advantage, some of which will also be reflected in increased resources, although many other measures of success exist.

THE HIV/AIDS URBAN ACTION NETWORK
IN NEW YORK CITY

The earliest writings and discourses on HIV/AIDS emphasized the social marginality and inherent "differences" of those who were affected by HIV/AIDS. The first wave of organizations struggled to gather and disseminate knowledge, among themselves and beyond. Most of this work may be considered the "pre-network" phase out of which the subsequent interorganizational field emerged. Although the early activists organized volunteer caregiving and invented the "buddy system" that is now part of the standard of community care for people living with HIV/AIDS, their most lasting accomplishments were definitional. Early community organizers changed the language of HIV/AIDS and established the social and political agenda that would dominate for the next decade and a half. They brought a new organizational field into being and defined the kinds of work that would be necessary in this field.

In the words of informants who were involved, AIDS work was a "blank slate in the early 80s." The earliest groups mobilized "anyone who knew something" about AIDS. This was a small group, but it created and relied upon connections across personal, professional, and subcultural boundaries, explicitly forming the base of what would become a vast network. As the field differentiated into more focused, more formally organized efforts, these early links created overlaps of interests, history, culture, and information exchange that lasted the lifespan of the network.

Once a field of work had been established, other organizers could define their goals in terms of the existing groups. The buyers' club Direct AIDS Alternative Information Resources (DAAIR), for example, sought to add a new voice and a new perspective to the variety of community-based HIV/AIDS work. Their development and integration into the existing network is an example of enrollment, as they strategically established connections with organizations in the empowerment arm of the field and formed a complementary relationship with the buyers' club People with AIDS (PWA) Health Group. A more explicit example occurred with the formation of the Haitian Coalition of AIDS (HCA), which grew out of the organized Haitian community in Brooklyn but immediately sought educational resources from GMHC, which they translated into French and Creole. HCA's connection to GMHC formed one of the first interorganizational linkages out of which the network grew.

Organizational splits were more difficult to identify during the early years, when many groups were only loosely constituted. The founders of numerous groups, including the Community Health Project (CHP), the PWA Health Group, and the People with AIDS Coalition (PWAC), had roots in the New York AIDS Network, and some of their organizational preparation grew out of that forum. Materially, however, CHP required a reorientation of personnel and resources out of the older St. Marks' Place Clinic, which predated HIV/ AIDS. Body Positive was founded by some of the leaders of PWAC, but not as an offshoot of that group, and the Momentum Project grew out of a GMHC project, with active support from an existing service network at St. Peter's Church. Once PWAC had formed an organizational center for the HIV/AIDS empowerment movement in New York City, most of the subsequent groups in that area, including Friends in Deed and Body Positive, developed in that space. Many more organizational splits occurred during later stages of networking as the larger multifunction organizations such as ACT UP gave rise to various independent groups with specialized roles.

The growth and differentiation of the network was enabled by an increasing number of participants and a wider resource base for the field overall, but it was driven by the diversification of organized action and the constant redefinition of the needs of the community. The first wave of activity had identified services and access to medical care as crucial areas for community-based intervention. As the next wave began, CBOs concerned mostly with the service and treatment arms defined their missions more narrowly around those functions, while new groups took on harm reduction and other outreach for intravenous drugs users, access to experimental and alternative treatments, community-based clinical research, minority education and treatment, adolescent outreach and prevention, AIDS treatment and care for women, and touching on all of these, an empowerment movement for people with HIV/ AIDS. Although this period was marked by increasing specialization, it was also characterized by considerable overlaps of function and constituency, as well as a high degree of overlapping membership. The processes by which new concerns and new constituents were defined for community-based AIDS work were also the processes through which new organizational spaces were defined within the network, and, correspondingly, through which new interorganizational relations came into being.

Additional points of contact occurred where two CBOs serving different constituencies, adopting different tactics, or pursuing distinct goals discovered an overlap of their interests. The Minority Task Force on AIDS (MTFA), for example, included in its mission counseling and education on healthy living with HIV. For current and reliable nutritional information, they drew upon God's Love We Deliver (GLWD). GLWD itself had begun as a very small operation run out of the founder's kitchen. As the demographics of the disease changed, and as HIV/AIDS became more of a chronic condition requiring ongoing support, GLWD's mission also grew. Expansion brought them to the outer boroughs and into the political domain of services to underserved minority communities and hence into contact with organizations such as MTFA.

CONCLUSION: NETWORKS ARE CULTURAL

A field expands as new groups split off from the center, shooting out into uncharted territory. It consolidates as these groups forge ties with others in both the new and the old spaces. It remains coherent when the participants define themselves as part of a single process. Like an ethnic subculture or even a nation (B. Anderson 1991; Hall 1990), an organizational field functions as an entity because its members believe that it is an entity and are able to narrate a history that makes them one.

It is difficult to conceptualize the shared cultural histories of organizations. The shared experiences among individuals throughout a field of action contribute to it, as do the common political and social environments in which the groups operate. Individuals who have shared participation in a past campaign carry that experience into their later organizational activities (Meyer and Whittier 1994). But such personal effects are only tangentially related to the network processes under discussion. More importantly, the older campaign becomes part of the cultural history of the field itself (at least it does to the extent that individuals from the prior campaign identify current work as part of the same field of action, and if these former participants remain in the field). A field has a history as well as a structure (Lune and Martinez 1999). The configuration of organizations reveals lines of development and the history of the growth of the underlying movement. The field links organizational structures to forms of action, past and present. Ideas circulate. Priorities and meaning systems are debated, but not necessarily decided upon. These, too, consolidate or fail to consolidate. Through organized collective efforts, these ideas and priorities are translated into actions. Organizations, albeit of people, are the collective actors in this history.

NOTE

1. Unfortunately, I did not speak with Mr. Jones for this study. The description quoted was from another African American activist familiar with the organizational split.

Conclusion

In anticipation of the World Social Forum held in Porto Alegro in 2005, members of attending organizations were asked which "issues, problems, proposals or challenges" they wished to take up at the forum.[1] The question following that one read,

What kind of activity would be more appropriate to deal with these struggles, issues, problems, proposals or challenges?

( ) audiovisual
( ) celebration
( ) conference
( ) controversy
( ) demonstration
( ) dialogue
( ) march
( ) music
( ) newspaper/radio/TV/Web
( ) party
( ) panel
( ) poetry and narrative
( ) research
( ) seminar
( ) testimony
( ) theater
( ) visual arts
( ) workshop
( ) other. Describe.

The organizers and participants who created the HIV/AIDS field of work in New York City in the early 1980s gradually established a network of interorganizational relations among community-based organizations. This "urban action network" linked the local groups to one another in a fluid form. The form itself enabled rapid communication, the mobility of individuals throughout the field, and a means for coordinated growth without central control. It enabled, and even encouraged, groups in the network to expand their reach, to independently form new connections across state and city borders, across forms of action, and beyond the community level.

The organizational innovations deployed by the groups working in the field of HIV/AIDS were never entirely new. Many of the activists and organizers had prior experience with political activism or community-based work in the social services arena. They brought their knowledge to bear on the new problem of HIV/AIDS in the United States. Their accomplishment was a fiercely dynamic recombination of tools and techniques, a shifting patchwork of interorganizational relations, and an unrelenting campaign to change the "institutionalized" approach to AIDS. For many reasons, this popular mobilization rode the crest of a new wave of social activism, unique to its times. Their most creative accomplishments were not tactical but definitional. They elaborated a new spatial and temporal context for collective political contention. Underlying all that they did was a floating sense of the "space" of work. They were in a place, and of a place. Yet their domain was virtual, not in the sense of existing through the Internet, but in the sense that, like the Internet (and so much else at present), they acted and interacted in what Manuel Castells has called "the space of flows" (1999).

Breaking new ground, the organizers of the HIV/AIDS field eschewed the idea of having to choose a single set of tactics or to choose between seeking state support or protesting state policies. They rejected the notion that they had to move from one clearly defined set of tactics or one stated political posture to another. They let stuff happen. By protesting the perceived lack of leadership at the state level, the community organizers demanded more government action while also insisting on their own right to be a part of that process. They created a new agenda for the state, attacked the old one, and simultaneously lent their support to allies within the state institutions who might champion the change. Far from being discredited or disenfranchised by their association with the activists, the advocates and service providers who spoke the language of industry and government were empowered and defended by them. The "good community activists" were invited to join the process in part because state actors wanted to keep the "bad community activists" away. The fact that many of the new insiders were former outsiders was not a problem for them or their state-based partners. Anything that expanded the boundaries of the field strengthened the network.

The years in which the HIV/AIDS field grew, from the early 1980s to the early 1990s, also witnessed vast changes in communications and travel technologies, the opening of national borders, and vast shifts in the power dynamics between states and citizens throughout much of the world. People and money moved rapidly. Data, including HIV clinical data, flew from its most obscure sources to a massively diverse global audience, bypassing the normal gatekeepers of scientific discourse (Epstein 1996). In this context, both community organizers and state officials had to adapt new forms of acting and interacting. These patterns of interaction have themselves now become part of the standard repertoire of political contention. As demonstrated in the World Social Forum's "thematic consultation form" quoted above, a loose and open assortment of forms of collective action are now not only expected within a single event but are actively encouraged. There is less concern with forming a single "unified" message and more support for the boisterous multitude.

Does multivocality still produce results? The activist Starhawk, in an essay she wrote within a few days of being released from a Seattle jail following the famous 1999 protests, suggested that the police there "were unprepared for the nonviolence and the numbers and commitment of activists—even though the blockade was organized in open, public meetings and there was nothing secret about our strategy" (2002, 52). The media coverage of the Seattle protests were, like the event itself, far more extensive than anyone had expected and much less casually accepting of the corporate version of events than usual. Despite the widespread focus on the broken McDonald's windows, press coverage also started to report on the activists' concerns. Neither the police nor the World Trade Organization (WTO) event organizers were able to contain or adjust to the massive activist blockade. The action itself involved a coalition of labor groups and environmentalists ("teamsters and turtles," as they became known); immigration rights groups; human rights groups; and many others. It was the coalition effect itself, according to Starhawk, that empowered the activists and outflanked the police.

My suspicion is that our model of organizing and decision-making was so foreign to their picture of what constitutes leadership that they literally could not see what was going on in front of them. When authoritarians think about leadership, the picture in their minds is of one person, usually a guy, or a small group standing up and telling other people what to do. Power is centralized and requires obedience. In contrast, our model of power was decentralized, and leadership was invested in the group as a whole. People were empowered to make their own decisions, and the centralized structures were for coordination, not control. As a result, we had great flexibility and resilience, and many people were inspired to acts of courage they could never have been ordered to do.

In the years since the "Battle of Seattle," the conflict between the transnational agencies of globalization and the global justice movement has simmered down some. The WTO and others have blunted some of the activist edge by accepting some of their demands. In 2005, for the first time in its ten-year history, the World Trade Organization invited outsiders to participate in the selection of its new director general. And while the participation did not include the right to vote, seventy labor, environmental, and "anti-WTO" activists were among those able to question the candidates in an unusually public forum. As well, representatives from many of the organizations in the global justice movement participated legitimately in other aspects of the World Economic Forum (WEF) summit meetings in Davos, Switzerland, at the end of January 2005. This was not the original strategy of the WEF, which, since 1999, had been avoiding the world's major cities for their annual meetings in favor of more remote and expensive sites. The *Los Angeles Times*'s coverage may have credited the corporations rather than the activists with the "new" strategy of incorporation, but their headline highlighted the distance that the protesters have traveled: "From the Streets to the Inner Sanctum" (Iritani 2005).

Nonunified Field Theory

In order to make sense of the case of HIV/AIDS organizing in New York City, I have relied on two distinct but related spatial concepts: networks and fields. To conclude this study, I will return to the questions with which I began this research. In discussing the answers that I propose, I use the case study that I have presented to identify several implications, both practical and theoretical, for the study of urban action networks and future variants on the form. Most of the discussion that follows will therefore concern the nature of organizational fields and interorganizational networks and the relevant attributes of each as they relate to one another. To this point I have focused on community-defining and community-building efforts and the role of community-based nonprofit organizations (CBOs). In order to generalize this conclusion, however, I adopt the broader language of nonprofit organizations (NPOs) and the relations of the nonprofit sector with the state.

We can view an organizational field as a shared space of work, a place in which social actors interact and where collective action and collective identity are negotiated. This interpretation follows indirectly from Paul DiMaggio and Walter Powell's proposition that "highly structured organizational fields provide a context in which individual efforts to deal rationally with uncertainty and constraint often lead, in the aggregate, to homogeneity in structure, culture and output" (1983, 148). Although their approach to the subject was broad and multifaceted, in this statement the authors were emphasizing commercial fields and the decisions of corporate leaders, conditions in which homogeneity is highly valued and diversity increases market uncertainty. Nonetheless, in that and subsequent works (e.g., Powell 1991), they provide room to consider other forms of interaction with less internal competition and more opportunities for heterogeneity. Even in the earlier, more restricted formulation, the processes leading toward homogeneity involve a gradual, negotiated convergence based on (unequal) input from all of the participants in the field.

Looking at fields spatially, we can observe that the relations among the different groups depend on their "locations" within the field. In previous studies, location has most often been predetermined and fixed. When DiMaggio (1991, 267) observed that "[field] structuration processes are historically and logically prior" to, among other things, the institutional processes that help to routinize the relationships among the organizations that constitute the field, it was clear that the corporations, foundations, academic institutions, and government bodies in his study occupied relatively fixed relations to one another in what had once been an emerging field, in this case American art museums. The question was how these structured relations would facilitate the negotiation of a new institution. The new field was built by a predefined set of social actors, each with established histories, connections, and patterns of behavior. The field was constructed through the elaboration of new relations in a new space.

The relatively fixed locations and predefined forms and identities of past cases yielded an interesting set of temporal relations. A lot of things were able to happen concurrently even though they were interdependent. The social actors of the field, in the case of fine art museums and in other cases, were or became so well known to one another, so interconnected, and so basically predictable to one another that one did not have to wait for one stage of some action to occur before the next would respond to it. After all, the shared goal underlying the routinization of relations in a field is to reduce uncertainty. The field defined both the spaces in which each party was free to act and the spaces and actions that were more constrained. The shared assumptions of the actors in the field allowed them to behave in ways that confound causal analysis by responding to the anticipation of an act before the act has been realized. The homogeneity of the field did not mean that they all looked alike or acted alike, but that they all adopted a more-or-less shared sense of how each role in the field was to be enacted. Everyone who did the same job did it in a comparable manner, and others could almost take that for granted.

In this sense, a newly emerging field creates new temporal relations as well as spatial ones. As long as the participants—nonprofit organizations in the case of HIV/AIDS—recognize their interdependencies and those interdependencies are not hierarchical, then the need to share information may be greater than the benefits of sharing any other resources. They cannot control one another, but they need to anticipate each other. Predictability within the field is crucial.

In business and in government, predictability beyond the field is also essential, because it supports the process of building external relations. In business and in government, the assumption is that relations are mutually beneficial. Within social movement studies, some models have attempted to incorporate both friendly and hostile relations within a single "multiorganizational field" (Klandermans 1992). Most often, however, a field does not need to deal with hostile interorganizational relations. Instead, it deals with competition, as multiple actors (individual, group, corporate) vie for control over a set of relations or exchanges. The competition is within the field; strictly speaking, it is within or around a single location in the field. The locations being relatively fixed, the competition is over who can best occupy the role.

Multiple forms of organizations may be found within any single policy domain, pursuing a complex array of channels into the policy process (Pizzorno 1987). In fields that incorporate nonprofit organizations acting in areas focused on state agencies, the structure of the field will reflect the relations between the organizations as well as the relations of the NPOs to the state (Caniglia 2001). Organizing activities take place within the field and are thus defined in relation to the configuration of relations throughout that field. The constraints and opportunities inherent in a nonprofit organization's location within the state-nonprofit system of relations guide the organizational forms and actions chosen by different NPOs (Diani 2001). The choice by one organization to specialize in a particular mission frees the others from responsibility for work in that area. One may walk softly while another carries a big stick.

ORGANIZATIONAL INNOVATION

One of the unique features of the present case is that most of the preexisting organizations and institutions that should have occupied clear locations in the HIV/AIDS field chose not to take their places. Had government, the public health sector, and the pharmaceutical industry treated this case as less exceptional, the field of HIV/AIDS work would likely have required a minor reshuffling of the usual players. Instead, the field began as an absence, a void that needed to be filled, which was then filled largely by new organizations. For this reason, the groups had first to commit to their individual missions and identify the types of relations necessary to serve those missions before they could enter into specific debates over the nature of the field itself. Yet these missions were themselves defined in relation to shared notions of what the field was and should be. Philosophy and strategy, structure and action, more or less coincided.

As a field defines and delimits a space of work, it gives structure to the plausible forms of relations within that space. Externally, or at the institutional level, a field of work is a "recognized" domain in which something "routinely" occurs (DiMaggio and Powell 1983). Internally, it is the proximate environment in which organizations operate. And that environment is composed of, among other things, a network of interorganizational relations through which certain roles are enacted. In an established field, the various roles will be institutionalized—familiar, taken for granted, and somewhat rigid. In a newly emerging field, the roles and the relations among them will be more open to interpretation and negotiation. Certain roles and relations might emerge quickly based on tradition, previous experience, or copying from other fields. Many will not. This provides, if only temporarily, an enhanced opportunity for organizational entrepreneurship.

The HIV/AIDS field, as it emerged, had unique amounts of slack from the outside hostile elements within its domain and almost no recognized organizational history to draw upon. If the museum field had opened out like a planned city (recalling that planned cities necessarily involve a lot of fighting before a plan takes shape), then the HIV/AIDS field was Deadwood. There was no plan, no sheriff, and no preferred form. Yet, as the field grew, the relations among the participants consolidated. Even as their relations with outside agencies became increasingly complex, their internal relations followed a familiar dynamic. The field took shape. Constant coordination accompanied their diversity. Their shared goals and nonprofit status greatly diminished the usual incentives for internal competition, so they didn't need to fight for control of individual roles. They were able to divide the labor because there were continuous discussions going on about what that labor should be, and there was more than enough "room" for everyone.

How did the diversity of the field serve the collective interests of the participants? To begin with, there could have been no collective purpose without it. With so many interests and issues at stake, a single strategy would have been unfeasible (MacNair, Fowler, and Harris 2000). Given the degree of uncertainty surrounding all HIV/AIDS issues during the first decade and the rate of change of both the epidemic and the state of our knowledge, a single "master frame" (Benford 1993) would have become obsolete too quickly. More to the point, the participants had little choice but to maintain a decentralized system of coordination if they were to coordinate at all. Despite the inequality of resources throughout the field, no single group or local community had the means to bring the rest into a form of action not of their own design. And despite the prominence of certain groups in particular subfields of work, the participants' descriptions of their individual careers in the field and of the interorganizational relations they cultivated indicate a considerable mobility of personnel, information, and material resources. That is, they shared.

The network was multivocal, open, and flexible—but not equal. There were complaints and competition, but there was room for that. Indeed, the frequency with which the groups chose to coordinate increased opportunities for conflict, which has been shown to be a routine part of voluntary alliances (York and Zychlinski 1996). With no fixed resource dependencies prior to the formal involvement of government, inequality was less of a threat to the survival of individual organizations. Coalitions, partnerships, and coordinated events came and went rapidly with few attempts to maintain the regular structures on which they relied other than for grant-related purposes. Interestingly, the growth and functioning of the network would probably have been more threatened by a large number of successful attempts at coalition formation than by a large number of failures. The lack of formality of the interorganizational ties allowed the organizations to remain innovative across the years.

Strength through Diversity

Changing relations between state agencies and organized communities are often conceptualized as a gradual, even inevitable course toward "professionalization" (Kleidman 1994; Zald and McCarthy 1987) and "routinization" (Michels 1968; Weber 1978), or more generally, "institutionalization" (McCarthy, Britt, and Wolfson 1991; Minkoff 1994; Oliver 1991). Each of these related processes has in common a single assumption, that community groups will, one way or another, have to change their organizational forms from whatever it is they originally wanted toward something more bureaucratic, more stable, and more compatible with the state or other institutional actors. Institutionalization tends to increase a community group's perceived legitimacy while decreasing its influence. As so many groups change from so many different forms into minor variations on the same form, agency at the local level is greatly diminished. It hardly matters how many social actors are involved in a conflict if they all act in the same way and through the same channels.

The processes of institutionalization have been observed many times among individual organizations or social movements. It's a solid thesis. Yet, while the idea may well describe the effects of a well-ordered field on a single organization in the field, it does not seem to speak as well to the effect of environments on entire fields. Even if someone somewhere in the field is pressured into adopting a bureaucratic hierarchy or redefining its mission, that doesn't mean that everyone in the field has to do the same. In fact, the institutionalization of some may well function as a buffer for the rest.

The diversity of the HIV/AIDS field appears to have provided such a buffer effect. The flexibility of the urban action network enabled the local groups to maintain their uniqueness and hence their individual voices in the web of state-community relations. As we have seen, different groups working with or against the same state agencies on the same issues were able to take contradictory positions without constraining one another's efforts. On the contrary, the fact that individuals with multiple group affiliations simultaneously participated in these seemingly opposing actions demonstrates that community organizers were aware of the value of this division of labor. Robert Wachter (1991, 131–32) observed exactly this strategy at work during the preparations for the 1989 International Conference on AIDS:

> Paul Boneberg [from the San Francisco CBO Mobilization against AIDS] sent a letter . . . to AIDS advocacy and activist groups all over America in defense of the conference. . . . Boneberg [also] warned us of the fragility of the activists' support and the possibility of disruptions if we weren't more forthcoming on free passes to the conference for people with AIDS. "Let me understand you," Dana [a conference staffer] said to Boneberg. "The conference is very important, and you want to preserve it. However, if you succeed in preserving it, then you may spend most of your time there disrupting it." "Yeah, that's about right," said Boneberg.

What was the value of this dual strategy? At least two results stand out. The first, as mentioned above, was that the community was able to resist institutionalization for a considerable period of time. The observed tendency for some community organizations to alter their organizational forms or to choose state-friendly forms in the first place provides evidence for the state's influence over the actions of private organizations in the "independent sector" (Jenkins and Eckert 1986; Smith and Lipsky 1993;Wolch 1990). This introduces the second apparent result of the community's organizing strategies. The freedoms afforded to the rest of the field, buffered by the state-friendly groups that were always among the most visible wings, limited the ability of state agencies to exercise influence over the rest of the field. By extension, the discourses, priorities, and values of the field as a collective were relatively independent of outside influence. Before the state could establish working partnerships with community groups, therefore, the relevant state agencies had to accommodate their forms to those of the organized community (Arno and Feiden 1992; M. Brown 1997; Epstein 1996). Although this result was not without precedent (Bordt 1997), it had not seemed at all likely for most of the 1980s (Wolfe 1997).

It is highly implausible that the field of nonprofit, community-based organizations working on HIV/AIDS issues simply became powerful enough to alter the state's priorities and actions, but it is equally unlikely that government agencies just "came around" after a while because it was the right thing to do. The work of the community groups gave public meaning to HIV/AIDS, even over the din of hate radio, homophobic campaigns, abstinence-only sex education, and a media discourse that contained a considerable amount of fear and alienation. HIV/AIDS was repackaged. Through appeals and threats, marches and workshops, art and international conferences, the field got its message(s) out. Once the public perspective on HIV/AIDS began to normalize and medicalize and once the national and international field of public health prominently took up both the challenge of HIV and the support offered by the organized community, the state began to look negligent for its strange silence. They had, therefore, to join a conversation that was already very much in progress.

The groups in question have had many successes and many failures across the years. On balance, however, their accomplishments have been amazing. HIV/AIDS prevention education has been institutionalized within grade school curricula throughout the nation along lines that were initiated by community groups. Most HIV/AIDS service organizations are now primarily supported by public funding. Older advocacy movements in other areas have begun to emulate HIV/AIDS groups (Anglin 1997), and researchers throughout the public health sector have sought partnerships with the affected communities. Syringe exchange programs are hardly even controversial anymore (Kelley, Lune, and Murphy 2005). Such pragmatic changes would not have been conceivable without significant cultural shifts, and these, too, reflect the efforts of the organized HIV/AIDS community. HIV/AIDS was once anathema to all political discussions, with the exception of the occasional antigay polemics that used it as a source of fear and marginalization. Now even figures like Jesse Helms, once a leading polemicist against all things AIDS-related, could call for increased government spending on HIV prevention and care. All of this must be credited to the actions of a community of people who, when they started, were sick; scared; displaced from jobs, homes, and families; and generally more hated than ignored (MacKinnon 1992).

Jesse Helms himself might have disagreed with this conclusion. Following years of aggressively blocking funding for HIV/AIDS in Congress and opposing foreign aid on most nonmilitary matters, Helms's proposal for increased foreign aid on HIV was one of his last campaigns before his retirement in 2003. Helms, one of the activist community's most reviled targets,[2] attributed his conversion to the efforts of Bono, the lead singer from U2, rather than to anything related to the activism or lobbying efforts of the organized community (Sandalow 2002). Yet it is unlikely that even Bono could have effected such a change without Helms's prior exposure to thousands of events and accusations throughout the years, many of which addressed him personally and vitriolically. Some sort of cultural conversion had to precede his personal epiphany. That was the discursive accomplishment of the field's multivocality.

CULTURAL POLITICS OF THE CITY

Why was collective action in the HIV/AIDS field so diverse for so long? There are multiple reasons, some of which are specific to the temporal and geographic details of this case, and some of which appear to be more general phenomena. Nonprofit efforts often proliferate where communities perceive that the state has "failed" to meet its responsibilities to the public or to select portions of the public (James 1987; Weisbrod 1988). But it was important as well in this case that the physical space of organizing contained so many distinct social communities, each improvising its own response. It is common to describe cities as "multicultural," as though the multiple collective identities implied by the term were merging and integrating. In practical terms, however, as Akhil Gupta and James Ferguson (1991, 7) have observed, we still have a great deal of difficulty separating identity and culture from places, both conceptually and experientially. People sometimes refer to "the culture" (singular) of Chicago, or of the United States, or even of Asia, rather than "the cultures" of those places. In "the city," where cultures and groups constantly collide, where "strangers are likely to meet routinely" (Sennett 1992, 128), patterns of interaction are in an ongoing state of renegotiation.

New York City is both large and crowded. Without a density of social actors—without a large city—there could not have been such a broad community mobilization as we find in the case of HIV/AIDS. The extended period of institutional avoidance, the "slack," allowed the period of organizational entrepreneurship to continue far longer than even the participants expected, leading to a consistently reported realization throughout the field that the community groups had both more power and more responsibility to make the organizational decisions for the field on behalf of "their own people." But all the while, the question of who belonged to which people remained open.

Earlier, I identified the three preconditions of the urban action network form as novelty, slack, and scope. The mobilization and remobilization of local communities in New York was a local adaptation to a normal, necessary process for a new field. They were doing what groups do with the mix of resources and needs that one finds in urban movements under conditions of crisis. They started new groups, pressed new claims, and looked to the city and the state for a response. The space they shared was physical more than organizational. Most of the early-riser organizations met within walking distance of one another. The fact that the external conditions failed to follow a more standard form reflected back on the work of the organized communities. Having failed to be co-opted by the city, the groups expanded their missions, took on new responsibilities, and looked for new targets. New situations occur; novelty plus slack engenders greater innovation.

The third component, scope, is also normal to some degree. In this case, the broad scope of the field was emphasized by the participants as a means for both expanding their recruitment and support possibilities and for encouraging diversity. This would have been even more important, but less clearly effective, for organizers in smaller cities with fewer HIV/AIDS cases and without the deep pool of activists and volunteers to draw upon. Strategically, there was no incentive for participants to limit the scope of the public's understanding of HIV/AIDS issues for the first ten years. Much of the early work was dedicated to "normalizing" AIDS and to resistance against the isolating and marginalizing rhetoric that was driving HIV/AIDS policy making at that time. It was only with the identification of HIV/AIDS as a serious national priority in the early 1990s, accompanied by a significant influx of public funding, that anyone had any reason to defend their ownership over any part of the field. Prior to that, both the general goals of the field and the specific goals of individual organizations were more often served by expanding the network. The increasing specialization of roles, coupled with the ongoing consolidation of interorganizational relations, added voices and other resources without introducing comparable constraints on their actions. In fact, diversification eventually became a key organizational strategy for overcoming the constraints inherent in particular roles and relations, as was demonstrated by some of the organizational splits.

Through coordinated interorganizational relations, the networked community groups in New York City were able to make a virtue of their disadvantages. They aggressively used their outsider status even as they actively pursued insider connections. They worked local politics and media as members of "the community" while spearheading a national and international mobilization. Such a combination of local and "displaced" activity exemplifies what Castells called "the new culture of cities . . . the culture of meaningful, interactive communication enacted by a multimodal interface between the space of flows and the space of places" (Castells 1999, 382). Some of this duality, with less coordination, was evident even within the first year of HIV/AIDS. By the time of the AIDS Coalition to Unleash Power (ACT UP), in the late 1980s, it was a routine. They did not have a relationship with government—they had many.

The urban action network model incorporates virtual connections and indefinite spaces, but it cannot work without a reasonably bounded physical space. Networked NPOs establish complex, informal coordination systems based on the rapid flow of information through many redundant links, some of them physical. Members meet, talk, and plan at the individual level as groups exchange information, refer people to one another, and just try to stay visible in their field. The groups' ability to coordinate, or at least to keep a close eye on one another and plan accordingly, is enhanced by coparticipation in small events of overlapping interest that bring groups with related concerns into frequent contact. Membership and leadership overlaps also assist community efforts to combine work when necessary and to reduce duplication of labor at other times, which also requires a shared physical world in which people can move from one group to the next. The publications that organizations distribute to their clients, members, and supporters as well as to each other further assist in the process of defining the boundaries around each group's role and around the different subfields of work while creating bridges across those boundaries. Yet the primary means by which the publications commingle, even in the Internet age, is simply by being stacked next to one another in waiting rooms and meeting spaces.

Decentralizing, Then Recentralizing, Power

"At their best," Arturo Escobar (2004, 210) recently wrote, "today's movements, particularly anti-globalisation and global justice movements, enact a novel logic of the social, based on self-organising meshworks and largely non-hierarchical structures. They tend to show emergent properties and complex adaptive behaviour that movements of the past, with their penchant for centralisation and hierarchy, were never able to manifest." They mix. They flow. They adapt. This logic is clearly both a form of interrelating among themselves and of dealing with institutions of power. Confronting power, being co-opted by it, or simply failing to gain influence are age-old concerns for collective actors. Confronting while also co-opting power through the use of complex "meshworks" is emerging as a variant. Is it a valuable new strategy made possible by virtuality and new communication models, or is it simply how diversity plays out in a larger field? I have argued that it is a strategy. To better understand the strategy, one must consider the place of the multiorganizational field in terms of a multilevel field of government structures such as the federated system of local and national governments in the United States, or the awkward placement of supranational bodies (such as the United Nations or WTO) "above" the nation-state in world politics.

There are real limits to the freedom of organizations acting within the sphere of the polity. The state may not be in charge, but it is a significant social actor in the processes defining the relations and division of labor in the kinds of fields with which this study is concerned. The processes described here depend on the nature of the relations between states and organized communities. All organizations are embedded in institutionalized fields of activity, or "structures of social relations" (Granovetter 1985, 481). State, market, and civil society are three particularly visible institutional contexts, and NPOs define themselves in relation to their institutional environments. An organization's identity is therefore understood contextually, just as an individual's or a community's identity can only be defined in terms of a host of cultural and social artifacts (Bourdieu 1990; White 1992). Organizational fields whose goals are defined in terms of political processes depend upon the actions of the state, which gives shape to the institutional environment (Jepperson 1991). NPOs in a shared field are thus structurally distant from but not wholly independent of the public agencies with which they interact. The community-based NPOs in this study, for example, commonly refer to themselves as "the community" to distinguish themselves from state and industry. It is because the community is still dependent on the state that they need to make this distinction. It acknowledges that the universe in which they work contains more than just themselves.

The HIV/AIDS action network in New York may have defined itself in contrast to "the state," as I have described it. But the institutional environment in which the network acted most of the time was defined by city government and to a lesser degree, state government. This appears to have also increased the amount of slack in the relations between the network and the nation-state. HIV/AIDS was a national crisis, so the city's role was relatively limited. The state Department of Health did form an AIDS Institute, collect data, and even fund service provision through both city agencies and community groups. So, personal animosity with the various mayors notwithstanding, the city was not as threatened by the organized community's actions as the federal government was. But most of the organizations in question were locally defined and did not depend on federal funding or oversight for many years. The "Group of Eight" monthly conference call that linked major service and advocacy groups in New York, Los Angeles, San Francisco, and Washington, D.C., was not a national umbrella organization. It was a coordination mechanism linking urban actors. By thinking nationally and acting locally, the groups shifted the "space" of work briefly into and then out of the national policy domain as the occasion arose. The resulting decentering of the relations between the field and the state contributed to its independence, and hence its growth.

The organizational field of HIV/AIDS work in New York City and beyond has grown considerably since 1991. But it is no longer structured as an urban action network. The loose, horizontal ties between groups operating on behalf of their local communities have been replaced by vertical ties linking communities to the state through contracts with both private and public organizations, including both nonprofits and for-profit corporations. Some of the community-based nonprofits have chosen not to participate in the new system of relations, and some were never invited to. The professionalization and institutionalization of many of the groups is not surprising (Jenkins and Eckert 1986). But this process primarily reflects changes at the institutional level. Organizations respond to shifting opportunities and constraints in the environment in which they are embedded (Tolbert and Zucker 1983), and the availability of routine funding streams has fundamentally reoriented the field (Chambré 1996). The changes in the organizational forms of the HIV/AIDS groups, and related changes in the form of the network itself, were not driven by unspecified "life-cycle" shifts or ideological reevaluations. The community groups maintained and supported their informal network structure as a means to gain influence in the public policy sector. Abandoning this form was the price of admission to the new system, the one they had originally sought.

THE TRANSNATIONALIZATION OF THE URBAN ACTION NETWORK FORM

Globalization's "promise," or threat, to render the state obsolete has proven no more true than its promise to usher in a new era of global prosperity (Evans 1997), but it has greatly diminished the effectiveness of many state-centered forms of political engagement. The stakeholders in the globalization process cannot be limited to a single community of anything, nor perhaps limited in any other way. By name and design, the vast wave of changes working through the global economy affect everybody, though not equally, of course. The sites in which the processes are managed are mostly supranational bodies whose work is carried out in the space of flows, linked as much by e-mail and websites as by any physical event, touching down once each year in one or another city for a round of increasingly controversial talks.

Where, then, is the site of resistance? How is it organized? Whom does it target? As to the first point, resistance to globalization follows the "displaced" nature of global economic restructuring itself. Virginia Vargas, for example, argues that "the logic of globalization thus expresses itself within the social movements. If national politics are predetermined by what is decided at the international level, it is at this level that protests, and alternative projects, must also develop" (2003, 908). And while "the international level" is not inherently a place, neither is it unreachable. Increasing numbers of authors have, in fact, located the key events of globalization within networks of cities (Abrahamson 2004; Sassen 1994). Considerable amounts of what we term globalization occur not in supranational bodies reaching down from above but in urban areas reaching out beyond their regions and states to tie into the accelerating flow (Gottman 1989).

Just as globalization "happens" through the links among cities, social movement scholars have found movement organizations to be forming comparable links through which to contend in a transnational polity. Latin American regional feminism, for example, "can now more aptly be characterized as an expansive, polycentric, heterogeneous *field of action* that spans into a vast array of cultural, social, and political arenas" (Alvarez 1998, 295; emphasis in original). These fields bring multiple interests and collective actors into multiple polities simultaneously. "National and regional issue-specific networks (or 'identity' networks), also largely articulated by feminist NGOs—linking Black women's organizations, indigenous women, lesbian rights advocates, socialist feminists, domestic workers, feminists in political parties, and individuals and groups working on issues ranging from feminist ecology to violence against women to reproductive rights—similarly have propagated in recent years" (Alvarez 1998, 309).

Both Sonia Alvarez and Vargas note that antiglobalization (global justice) activism relies on networks of otherwise unaligned interests, but they interpret this as having to do with the logic of globalization itself. This is true, and yet the point elides the earlier hints and manifestations of such necessarily fluid organizational forms in less globally politicized fields. It might be more apt to suggest that whatever combination of late capitalist, postmodern, or high-tech forces drove markets and economic policy from a dominant model of state-centered planning into a border-crossing reevaluation of such hallowed notions as trade and even sovereignty has also precipitated a change in how deindustrialized politics takes place. The transformations in forms of collective action that are now evident in struggles over globalization were already under way years before the "Battle of Seattle." Urban activism in the 1980s was as "place based" and yet delocalized as everything else in the world's "global cities."

Critical responses to the Seattle protests and other parts of the global justice movement suggested that the movement was undermined by a lack of "unity of vision and strategy." Yet, as Naomi Klein wondered, "even if we did manage to come up with a ten-point plan—brilliant in its clarity, elegant in its coherence, unified in its outlook—to whom, exactly, would we hand down these commandments?" (Klein 2002, 265). More generally, she asks, Why does one need to reorganize a loose gathering of different voices, issues, constituencies, and targets into a single movement at all? Klein's preferred model for either coordinating what she calls "the anticorporate movement" or describing recent actions is a "network of spokes and hubs" (2002, 267).

> Rather than present a coherent front, small units of activists surrounded their target from all directions. And rather than build elaborate national or international bureaucracies, temporary structures were thrown up instead: empty buildings were turned into "convergence centers," and independent media producers assembled impromptu activist news centers. The ad hoc coalitions behind these demonstrations frequently named themselves after the date of the planned event: J18, N30, A16 and, for the IMF [International Monetary Fund] meeting in Prague on September 26, 2000, S26. When these events are over, they leave virtually no trace behind, save for an archived website.

How do states understand and respond to extrainstitutional politics in the Internet age (in wired countries, anyway)? My simple contention is that a very considerable part of the interaction between "state" and "citizen" is mediated through interorganizational relations between "agencies" of the state and private associations. The state is huge, complex, and inconsistent but also centralized and formally controlled. Citizens and communities of citizens are more complex, more diverse, and not formally related at all. Between the two, as celebrated by Alexis de Tocqueville, studied by Max Weber and warned against by Alexander Hamilton, there is an intermediary layer of organized interests. Contemporary scholarship on the political and economic roles of this sector of activity call it "civil society," and many writers view it as the space in which democracy itself really happens or fails to happen (see Edwards, Foley, and Diani 2001; Salamon and Sokolowski 2004). It is in this layer of activity that the uncountable millions of individual wants coalesce into platforms, proposals, and demands. This is the space where institutions meet communities.

Early scholars of collective action asked "why" people participate in such actions. This has been answered many times (in many different ways). A better question for the moment is "how" public politics occur. To answer that question, we also need to ask "where" action takes place. In other words, to explore the means of collective action we must first ask about the locations of action. Given a broad definition of contentious politics and the collective process, What is the space of collective action? The answer cannot be found in any one physical space. Rather, the space of political contention is, in general terms, the field of work and, in particular, the interorganizational relations that bind the field into a network. For a locally based field with a significant political agenda, these interorganizational relations may be characterized as an urban action network.

NOTES

1. This form, which was available as a PDF on the WSF website, is no longer available online.

2. A flyer distributed at the funeral of writer and activist Vito Russo stated, "I believe with all my heart that Jesse Helms killed Vito Russo," and described Helms as having "the blood and flesh of dead dykes and fags dripping from his hands and mouth" (Crimp 1992, 3).

Afterword

One can learn a great deal about social and psychological phenomena by examining the problems one encounters in trying to study them.

—Melvin Kohn, "Doing Social Research under
Conditions of Radical Social Change:
The Biography of an Ongoing Research Project," 1993

Starting in the mid-1990s, I set out to map the network of HIV/AIDS community-based organizations in New York City with an idea to study organizational clustering and to define a useful measure of centrality and influence within a new interorganizational field. I undertook small case studies, each involving three or four interviews with key informants; content analysis of organizational literature; and participant observation in meetings and public events. My first six or eight cases centered on organizational functions and interorganizational connectedness.

I had hypothesized that clustering (tight pockets of routine exchange within a larger network) would follow from function, and that organizational functions (e.g., service provision, politics, health care, etc.) would relate to organizational forms (e.g., a highly centralized or loosely coordinated or a patchwork of small groups, etc.). I anticipated that each cluster of activity would contain its own little world of activity, with identifiable organizational norms and priorities, prominent groups and individuals, and that the interactions across subfield boundaries would have to be negotiated around the differences in priorities. That is, I expected that all of the service organizations would have a lot of contact with other service providers, advocates with advocates, and so on, and not a lot of routine contact across functional lines. I anticipated that different types of groups would "look"

different, act different, and have different organizational cultures that made
it easier for them to work with groups of the same type and harder to work
with others. This wasn't entirely wrong; rather, it was a model that exaggerated differences and assumed that cooperation, when it occurred, had to
be explained. My initial model presumed that the structure of the field predicted organizational characteristics (where a group was located in the field
would predict what the group was like). It also presumed that the field structure determined, to some measurable degree, the system of meanings and interpretations that would be at work within any given location. For a time I
experimented with an assortment of graphic mapping programs to represent
the "true structure" of the field. Over time, as I became more immersed in
the process, I began to feel that I was looking for data in all the wrong
places, that I was leaving out a layer of reality that superceded most of what
I was trying to measure. Eventually I came to realize that the structure was
not the real issue. Organizations interacted in a myriad of ways with little
regard for the similarity or even compatibility of their forms, their stated
missions, or their locations within the network.

Happily, I had chosen to start each interview with personal questions about
the background and "career" trajectory of each of my informants. What I
learned from that was that HIV/AIDS work was, for most of my informants,
a calling and not a career. They did not divide the field into separate categories of function. They did not argue over the "right way" to do what they
did. (At any rate, they didn't do those things with any regularity before 1991.)
Most of the people whom I interviewed or e-mailed back and forth with were
more like voluntary firefighters in an endless summer of wildfires. They went
where they were needed, and they stayed as long as they could.

In a relatively short time, two patterns emerged. The first was that almost
no one worked within only one group, or even one cluster (or subfield). Their
histories were full of stories of multiple, often simultaneous public identities:
service provider in the morning, "buddy" in the afternoon, and activist nights
and weekends, without ever "becoming" a service worker, a buddy, or an activist. All of these forms of action were available to them, and all were
deemed necessary.

The second pattern was that very few informants seemed able to tell me
about their own work without explaining about the shape, history, and nature
of the whole field. And while the details of these capsule histories did not always entirely agree with one another or with published accounts, the overall
flow had coherence. With minor variations, the informants shared the same
system of meaning. When enough people realized that something needed to
happen that wasn't already happening, they started a new organization.

Thus, by serendipity, I learned that there was something self-consciously holistic about the organization of the field itself. It functioned as a unit, albeit loosely. My research question changed to "How do they do that?" In other words, instead of studying how groups negotiated cooperation when they had to, I began to study how the field maintained and promulgated the expectation that groups would cooperate. How was it that major and minor shifts in the structure of the field could generate more consensus than conflict? Primarily, this became a question of how each organization defined itself, the field, and its role in the field. And since organizations don't literally define themselves, the issue was how people in the field came to define their collective missions in relation to everything that everyone else was doing.

From that point, I began to "collect" more organizations and to triangulate my data on each of the parts of the field by seeking as many perspectives as possible within them. Each interview included data on interorganizational relations and collaborations, so each round of data collection sent me to more groups, often within the same area of activity. I added new topics to my interviews pertaining to how each informant viewed the work of groups with which they did not have routine contact. And I revisited my content analysis to search out and code all instances in which one organization referred to the work of others. There were almost too many to count, and mostly positive and supportive, with little manifest indication of competition between the groups. (Competition existed, but it was mostly kept "backstage.") The coding scheme that emerged eventually coalesced into four categories of interorganizational relations: collaboration, including outreach and enrollment; referrals; origins, including splits; and sponsorship, including the exchange of material resources and personnel. Each interview centered on a single organization but emphasized that group's role within the larger field. In this way, I sought to view the field overall from as many vantage points as possible.

A third pattern became clear as my fieldwork progressed. "Older" informants, those that had been active since at least the mid-1980s, spoke of different waves of activity and different periods of HIV/AIDS. The 1980s and the 1990s were different worlds. "Newer" informants mostly had only entered the field in the nineties. The different groups' official histories (from newsletters and later websites) demonstrated the patterns in the founding dates of organizations along which the chapters are divided, with a particular spike in 1987. But clearly *something happened* in or around 1990. Not surprisingly, that something had to do with money. Once that piece of the puzzle fell into place, I realized that the story I was putting together had its own boundaries, from 1981 to 1991. Although I entered the field for the first time only a few years after that, my topic was already becoming historical.

GROUNDED THEORY

I had brought many false assumptions with me into the field, including the expectation that subfields would compete for dominance and that activist organizations would be "winning" in some circles and absent in others. I was quickly reeducated by my informants. I had also begun with a perspective on state-community relations that emphasized legal restrictions and challenges. This, too, turned out not to be significant. The key issues in people's lives and organized action at the time that most of them entered into work in this field were cultural first and either political or pragmatic second. They competed with the state, in its various forms, over the meaning of HIV/AIDS. My conclusion, that cultural constructions preceded and guided political campaigns, formed slowly. Similarly, although I had chosen to study nonprofits due in part to my interest in extrainstitutional organizing, I had started with measures of formal linkages. I only learned about the importance of informal interorganizational linkages within the field because the people with whom I spoke told me about that.

Grounded theory, as a research methodology, does not mean that you poke about in your research setting until you stumble across something interesting. It is an iterative process by which you prepare your ideas, go out into the field to investigate them, and then "exit" the field to reflect on what you have learned. One goal during the fieldwork, perhaps the most important one, is to learn from the participants their definitions of the world you are studying. The researcher's definitions are also useful, but they cannot take precedence over the participants' experiences and interpretations. After refining your thoughts, tweaking your measures, and identifying the questions that your fieldwork has raised, you go back for more. The researcher collaborates with the subject; the informants are the experts, but the researcher does the overarching theory part. In this way, you discover meaning rather than imposing it. Part of this collaboration has included returning to organizations where I had conducted research in order to present my findings. My audience at these presentations were research subjects, experts, and critics simultaneously. Their feedback was invaluable, if sometimes unnerving. I was constantly reminded that I remained an outsider to their work. Phrases like "what you have to understand is . . ." highlighted all of the things I was only starting to get.

One of the strengths of the grounded theory approach is that it allows and encourages you, as a researcher, to describe what you are doing, literally and metaphorically, while you are doing it. The data collection and the interpretation are not held distinct. In surprising ways, I found that giving meaning to the data was tied to giving meaning to the data collection process. I had been interested in the *liminal* state of being that many people living with HIV/ AIDS have expressed, what Victor Turner called a period of existing "betwixt and between" defined states. For example, people live with HIV, but having been diagnosed as HIV-positive, they are perceived and often feel as though they are under a death sentence. A profile of Bailey House even reported that an administrator there wanted to organize a resident softball team called "The Dead" (C. Brown 1992).

Early on, I realized that the organizations of the field are liminal in other ways, and that the connection is more than metaphorical. To form a group of and for people who are both marginal and disliked is to seek empowerment for a people who are brought together by their powerlessness. This creates uncertainties among them about how to even describe who they are or what they are doing.

The organizational identities were liminal at a more fundamental level as well. Organizations often "act" to preserve their own continuity. But many of these organizations were directed toward their own obsolescence. The organizers do the work they do because they feel that it is needed, and they identify strongly with this work. If they succeed, then they will not need to do that anymore. Since the money situation changed in 1991, it has become popular to talk about the "AIDS industry." I have even had conversations with people outside of the field who believe that the true goal of HIV/AIDS organizations is to keep infection rates high in order to keep the grant money flowing. Such a glib suggestion serves only to dismiss the work studied here. The oft-repeated desire of so many informants in this study was to put themselves out of business, to no longer be needed. They wanted to get back to their old lives, where they had better-paying jobs and could take time off. At the same time, their organizational successes reified certain identities and categories as "the AIDS community," of which they were a part. This created further complications for those who did not fit the categories but who belonged within the community. They, too, were in between classifications, struggling to open up the definitions rather than to fit within the existing system.

Liminality informed the framework through which I came to understand the events that I studied. Often, as well, it helped me to think about my own status as a researcher. When the data denied some aspect of my expectations but I had not yet found new meaning in it, I went through periods of gathering information without exactly knowing what the data were for. I felt like a detective pacing back and forth in the same empty alley, hoping a clue would show up. This was my own experience of liminality, which caused me no small amount of anxiety. Taking the lead once again from my informants, I forged on and eventually came out on solid ground again.

ORGANIZATIONAL ETHNOGRAPHY

The methodology I followed derived from what has been described as "urban ethnography." While noting that some great theoretical work has come from this method, Gerald Suttles (1976) also observed that researchers doing this often have difficulty attaching an identified conceptual framework to their studies. One reason for this is what he called "methodological opportunism, which tends to bring the field worker into confrontation with such a range of social contact that it is difficult for him [*sic*] to rely fully on normative conceptions that do not leave much latitude for variation" (Suttles 1976, 2). For example, when you enter a "deviant" field because it is interesting, because it is deviant, you have a lot of ready-made data to work with, but you are burdened already with the externally defined assumption that it is deviant. The systems of meanings and values that have already defined the field of study may actively oppose or deny the many perspectives of the various people in the field itself. So any predefined conceptual model is suspect.

Even where we are less opportunistic, our desire to learn how other people make sense of their own experiences competes with any theorizing we might do about those same experiences. If you start asking how people respond to change and how they cope with the unexpected, you end up collecting a lot of people's individual theories about how the (local) world works. The assumptions and priorities of these belief systems, then, become further data to help conceptualize and predict actions. But then you have to account for their theories in your theories. Some social change organizations, for example, might be confrontational because they perceive their targets as enemies. Others might become confrontational this week only because they have talked about it and have decided that the time is right for that sort of thing. The observable events are similar, but the meaning systems are distinct. Their different worldviews link certain groups or individuals while forming barriers between others. Any attempt to "lock in" the groups' perspectives with a single unchanging definition becomes a gross oversimplification. To form a more accurate picture, the researcher must treat the information as pieces of a puzzle that has multiple solutions. You can't assume too much about meanings or priorities prior to this process.

The HIV/AIDS field was not particularly well defined as a study site when I began this work, but there were enough predefined meaning systems associated with it to obscure any new research. As I noted in the first section, writings about "AIDS victims," "AIDS risk groups," "innocent victims," and even "AIDS junkies" created a variety of interpretive frames through which the writers could draw a line between themselves and their readers on one side and between people living with HIV/AIDS on the other. Each of these framing devices implied some causal connection between character and disease. (Among those who deny, or have denied, that HIV is the cause of AIDS, the term "dis-ease" is sometimes used to suggest that AIDS afflicts people who are psychosocially predisposed to fall victim to life-threatening conditions. See, for example, Hay 1984.) It had become conventional to approach HIV/AIDS as a study in deviant culture and I was occasionally called upon to explain why I didn't see it that way.

The advent of HIV as a topic of social science had a curious side effect in this regard. Homosexuality itself had been viewed and studied as a form of deviance for decades before gay activists in and out of the academy pressured the major professional associations, like the American Sociological Association (ASA), the American Psychological Association (APA), and the American Medical Association (AMA), to broaden their perspectives. The APA listed homosexuality as a mental disorder until 1973; the Defense Department may be alone in still categorizing it as such (Baldor 2006). Prior to this reclassification, studies of homosexuals or homosexuality hardly seemed to require any deeper purpose or thesis. Whether you called it deviance, pathology, or a social problem, the very existence of the topic justified attention. From the mid-1970s on, homosexuality seemed to be more like other topics. There were reasonable and interesting questions to ask about it, but simply putting "the gay man" under a microscope was not valid.[1] Suddenly, with the appearance of the "gay cancer," there was a mini-explosion of writing, scientific and otherwise, about the behavior of gay men. In this environment, my approach was unusual. I treated organizations created by and for gay men (and drug users, and immigrants, and sick people, etc.) as social and political actors, not as curiosities. I hope we've gotten over that, and that present-day readers will see this decision as obvious. At the time of my fieldwork, however, the most common question I was asked was why I was interested in these groups.

Urban ethnography is a way of understanding neighborhoods, that is, spatially and culturally related collections of people. Since my interest is in city-centered organizational fields—spatially and culturally related collections of groups—I chose to conduct an organizational ethnography. Up to this point, the term "organizational ethnography" has been used somewhat inconsistently but usually refers to some kind of "case study." That is, it is used to describe qualitative research within an organization that attends to the culture of the organization or some select group within it. While popular and useful among consultants, this approach has not found a solid place in organizational sociology (Hodson 1998). But in order for the concept to truly be useful, I think it must go beyond individual case studies. I have therefore appropriated the term to include not just the culture within an organization but also the organizational culture within which the organization lies. In other words, I use the term "organizational ethnography" to describe fieldwork that contextualizes organizational cultural measures within a defined field of organizations.

My fieldwork, following this conceptualization, had a number of interesting and unique features. First, since no single organization can give one a sufficiently broad view of the field, I conducted mini–case studies at many organizations. Second, the field I had chosen was newly emerging. Most of the significant past studies on the origins and growth of organizational fields have relied heavily on archival data (Baum 1995; DiMaggio 1991). In contrast, most of the pioneers of the New York HIV/AIDS field were still in New York when I began my work. Further, the identity of the field in question was not only still in flux but was very much a subject of debate and discussion within the field as I moved through it. Not to be too "opportunistic," but it was a rare thing to witness a collective identity in formation.

The case of HIV/AIDS was uniquely appropriate for a study of shared meanings and collective identity. The organizations studied here had three sizable challenges, all of which had to do with the problem of collective identity. They were organized against the impact of the medical condition, which necessitated a fight for control of the public identity of HIV. They were organized against the stigmas that threatened the lives of people affected by HIV/AIDS, which required acting against a world of negative imagery long associated with racial, economic, and sexual minorities. And they had to struggle for their own recognition as legitimate social actors in social, political, and medical domains. Other fields typically begin with some professional or cultural-historical identity in relation to which the participants can explain themselves. The HIV/AIDS groups were united only by their agreement around conceptual goals. All of their work, therefore, depended on how they dealt with the problem of the identity of the field that they were constructing. The interplay of relations and meanings that they created was not simply a by-product of some other task. It was what they did.

Studying an organizational field also begins with difficult definitional work. Unlike urban ethnographers who can identify the borders of the neighborhood they are entering, I had to "find" my field in order to enter it. I started with a small number of points of entry, and I followed the paths opened by each.

First, there were key locations. I started this research by walking into the Center on 13th Street and taking notes on which groups in that space were doing what in response to HIV/AIDS. Visiting again and again over the next few weeks, walking from floor to floor, I knocked on doors, attended meetings (with permission), collected flyers, and just "hung around" talking with people. From this one perspective, I began to map the contours of the field.

I repeated the same approach at other key locations, such as the offices of Gay Men's Health Crisis (GMHC) and the People with AIDS Coalition of New York (PWAC/NY), both of which were used by multiple other groups for meetings, and both of which distributed a great deal of community literature to their clients and participants. These physical centers were also networking centers, and so I quickly learned who was connected to whom via these few hubs.

The second point of entry was provided by public events. Whether rallies, protests, funerals, fundraisers, or educational seminars, most of the bigger public events were co-organized by at least two or three groups and were attended by "members" of a great many more. Each time I marched, I not only encountered unfamiliar groups, but I also had the opportunity to trace back the connections that brought each unique combination of groups together. I was thus initially surprised to find that the "phone tree" clustering did not conform to any of my formal network models, did not reflect the political postures of the participant organizations, and did not even demonstrate tight grouping by demographic characteristics. As discussed throughout this book, the key ties were provided either by personal connections among individuals or by the complex history of relations between groups that had loaned support to one another, split off from one another, or recruited each other for some earlier campaign.

The third point of entry was the one that most resembled a formal research design. Using my collections of flyers, service directories, care network directories, and *The Encyclopedia of Organizations*, I made lists of groups divided by primary functions: service providers, legal advocates, women's health organizations, and so on. I then phoned the organizations in each grouping and requested an appointment for a formal interview and site visit. In cases such as syringe exchange/harm reduction, the grouping was small enough that I could reasonably contact all of them. For categories like general case management, I had to limit myself to the first five or six.

Additional contacts came about through the interviews themselves, as informants either simply made me aware of areas of work that I had not yet come across, or they more forcefully insisted that my research would be flawed if I did not meet some particular individual or visit some specific group.

Finally, I employed participant observation. Most of this work occurred during the data analysis phase after my "regular" data collection had been completed. I attended a few community forums pertaining to needs assessments and budget priorities as a participant rather than as a silent observer. I volunteered to assist in the event preparation for one AIDS Coalition to Unleash Power (ACT UP) demonstration, in a Housing Works weekend of activities related to harm reduction, and in occasional envelope-stuffing shifts around town. And in a reversal of the relationship I had established with other informants, I joined the Treatment Action Group's Legislative Affairs Committee and the Coalition for Women's Choice in HIV Testing and Care under the assumption that they could use a sociologist. These periods of deeper involvement allowed me to discuss my findings with knowledgeable participants as I was writing them. Inevitably, this also meant that I allowed some participants the opportunity to color my thinking. Nonetheless, my findings and my interpretations are my own synthesis of what I learned in the field; no other contributor to this study used such a model. Fortunately, no one with whom I have spoken in the field found my conclusions implausible.

GAINING ACCESS VERSUS GOING NATIVE

I never felt that I had to struggle to keep my perspective "safe" from the influence of the highly charged, even zealous groups of people whom I studied. On the contrary, I enjoyed being there. I loved working alongside them. I did not march in rallies with a hidden notebook and camera. I just marched. The events mattered for their own sake. Later, of course, I did write out notes. I was not an observer "acting" as a participant. I was a participant, observing. But I was never really an insider.

From the outset, I had chosen to enter a field with which I was relatively unfamiliar. I have worked with social advocacy groups before, and I did not want to allow my personal history to impair my research. At the same time, I wanted to be comfortable as a participant observer. It was important to me that my research could have some benefit, however transitory, to the people whose work I was studying. Whether the benefits would be limited to the few hours of volunteer work I did for some group one afternoon or as expansive as my finding something that could strengthen the work of the whole field, I wanted to feel that I had something to offer. I wanted to collaborate, in some form, with the subjects on their work, just as I had asked them to collaborate with me on mine. There are organizations out there for which I could not volunteer my time in good conscience, just as there are events and activities to which I could not gain access without deceiving people. By entering the HIV/AIDS field, I did not have to confront those problems. I was able to tell informants that I respected what they were doing and that I would treat the data they gave me with respect. Beyond that, I felt that the community-based field of mostly voluntary HIV/AIDS work was simply one of the most important "indigenous" social phenomena happening in the city at the time, and I wanted to be there.

We speak of fieldwork "capture," or "going native," as a threat to the validity of field research. A researcher who overidentifies with the subject loses objectivity. One who develops too much of an insider perspective gives up the alien's viewpoint that we value as properly scientific, though as I try to teach my students, that doesn't mean that researchers don't have perspectives or values. If we had no values at all, it doesn't seem likely that we would have any reason to study social phenomena. Of course, there are limits. You can't study things like movement-countermovement dynamics if you're convinced already that one side is right and the other wrong. A standard question, then, is how do we balance the desire to see things as our subjects see them with our desire to remain "objective"? I cannot help but rephrase the question: Can we trust a researcher who spends years among people who are ill or dying, among their networks of support and care, and among the industries and politics surrounding them and then claims to have had no personal feelings about the topic?

In this work, I sought to accomplish one of the things that I have described the groups themselves as having accomplished. I started as an outsider and worked to develop credibility as a kind of insider without actually surrendering my autonomy or my right to make my own judgments. I began from a position of sympathy and moved toward a position of empathy. I think I succeeded to a reasonable extent. But to be perfectly honest, I could not have become so enmeshed as to threaten my attachment to my professional detachment. Watching *Cape Fear* with a group of underemployed, underhoused African American injecting drug users can be a lot of fun for an employed White sociologist, but it doesn't magically break down cultural barriers.

There were many advantages to this approach, most of them having to do with shifting my attention from the structure of the field to its collective identity. First, I got to spend a lot of time with a lot of people doing "frontline" work in the HIV/AIDS field in New York. In this way, I believe I cut through the formal mission statements and programmatic language that organizations have to write about themselves and could see what people were actually doing. This kind of fieldwork also brought me into regular contact with people living with HIV/AIDS, the people around whom the field is supposed to be organized. Just as one can study governments and government policy without mentioning citizens, or industries without encountering consumers, it would be dangerously easy to study social service and advocacy groups without any unmediated contact with clients (or participants, members, or constituents, depending on the organization). Such contact, which some informants called a "reality check," tempers the academic habit of reducing everyone and everything to data.

I conducted formal interviews, from which most of the data derive. But I also participated in conversations over the meaning of the work that my sources were performing. I sat in on and contributed to strategy sessions in which participants distinguished among what they wanted to do, how it would be perceived by their communities, how it could be represented by the media, how it would be received by other groups, and how it should be explained to funders. These conversations helped me to interpret the ways in which participants in the field perceived the field, judged its gaps, and sought to alter its nature. They gave me glimpses into the minds of the organizers.

There were drawbacks as well. One obvious limitation is that I could only interpret the field through the perspectives of the people who spent time talking with me. I can't really say what the other participants thought, but of course everyone has their own stories. Nonetheless, as noted in the text, I encountered a lot of thematic consistency from one interview to the next and a great many supporting comments, written and spoken, throughout the research process. I have noted significant disagreements, where they occurred. Another limitation is that, as an outsider to the development of the field, I did not have the expert knowledge to protect myself against all errors. In preparing this text, I have found errors. Some of these may have come from my sources. Some were simply my mistakes. Fortunately, I have also had help from reviewers and other readers that made it possible to correct these mistakes and misperceptions.

ACKNOWLEDGMENTS

Various reviewers, anonymous and otherwise, have helped me to bring this work to completion. Other friends and colleagues have read large portions of earlier drafts and offered extensive advice and commentary. Particular thanks are due to John G. Dale, Hillary Oberstein, Paul Galotowitch, Miranda Martinez, Wolf Heydebrand, and Susan Chambré. I could not have finished the book at all without the support of my partner, Maureen Cummins. It is, however, the informants themselves who have made this work possible. Overworked, underpaid, and sometimes fighting for their lives, scores of activists, organizers, writers, and volunteers invited me into their world and took the time to teach me what I needed to know. I am grateful to them for their collaboration.

NOTE

1. My suggestion here is impressionistic, not measured.

Appendix A

Organizations Contributing to the Study

CBO	Primary functions[1]	Primary target population(s)	Region[2]
AIDS Coalition to Unleash Power (ACT UP)	Political activism	N/A	
AIDS Community Research Initiative of America (ACRIA)	Research, treatment education	N/A	
AIDS Service Center of Queens County (ACQC)	Case management, harm reduction, advocacy, mental health	PLWHIV/AIDS (people living with HIV/AIDS) and their families	Queens
AIDS Service Center of Lower Manhattan (ASC)	Case management	PLWHIV/AIDS	Manhattan
Alianza Dominicana	Counseling	Latino PLWHIV/AIDS and their families	Upper Manhattan and surrounding areas
Asian and Pacific Islander Coalition on HIV/AIDS (APICHA)	Case management, advocacy	Asian PLWHIV/AIDS	Citywide
Association for Drug Abuse Prevention and Treatment (ADAPT)	Harm reduction, related support	HIV-positive drug users	Brooklyn, Manhattan
AIDS Resource Center/Bailey House (ARC)	Case management, housing, technical assistance for HIV/AIDS service providers	Underhoused and homeless PLWHIV/AIDS and their families	Citywide
Body Positive (BP)	Information and support	PLWHIV/AIDS	Citywide
Brooklyn AIDS Task Force (BATF)	Case management, harm reduction, technical assistance to service providers, substance treatment	HIV-positive individuals in drug recovery, clients transitioning from COBRA	Citywide

Organization	Primary Services	Target Population	Region
Center for Community Alternatives (CCA)	Harm reduction, buddy services, limited case management	HIV-positive individuals involved with the criminal justice system	Citywide
CitiWide Harm Reduction	Harm reduction	Drug users and their families	Citywide
Coalition for Women's Choice in HIV Testing and Care	Advocacy	N/A	Citywide
Community Health Project/ Callen-Lorde Community Health Center (CHP)	Mental health services, medical care, case management	Uninsured HIV-positive individuals	Citywide
Broadway Cares/Equity Fights AIDS (BC/EFA)	Grants to service organizations	CBOs	Citywide
Direct AIDS Alternative Information Resources (DAAIR)	Buyer's club	PLWHIV/AIDS	Citywide
Exponents	Harm reduction, case management	HIV-positive individuals transitioning from Rikers Island Correctional Facility, active and recovering drug and alcohol users	Citywide
Friends in Deed (FID)	Counseling, support, nutrition	Anyone with a life-threatening illness, their families and friends	Citywide
Foundation for Research of Sexually Transmitted Diseases (FROST'D)	Harm reduction, recovery readiness, counseling	Active and recovering drug and alcohol users	Bronx, Brooklyn, Manhattan, Queens
Gay Men of African Descent (GMAD)	Services and support	GLBT (gay, lesbian, bisexual, and transgender) people of color	Citywide

(continued)

1. In some cases, depending on organizational literature, "primary" is a judgment call. Some of these organizations have changed their emphasis since the time of this research. Some are defunct.

2. The region designation indicates whether the organizations target a portion of the city or not. The designation "Citywide" also includes those groups whose reach is well beyond the city. No region is given for political, media, or research organizations that do not have clients, patients, or members.

CBO	Primary functions	Primary target population(s)	Region
Gay Men's Health Crisis (GMHC)	Case management, buddy services, advocacy, harm reduction, daily living assistance, counseling, treatment education	PLWHIV/AIDS and their families	Citywide
God's Love We Deliver (GLWD)	Food and nutrition	PLWHIV/AIDS	Citywide
Haitian Coalition on AIDS/ Haitian Centers Council (HCA)	Case management, housing referrals	Haitian PLWHIV/AIDS	Citywide
Harlem United Community AIDS Center (HU)	Case management, counseling, food and nutrition	Residents of East Harlem	Harlem section of Manhattan
Health Education AIDS Liaison (HEAL)	Information, support	PLWHIV/AIDS	Citywide
Hispanic AIDS Forum (HAF)	Treatment education, NYC-Puerto Rico transitional case management	Latino PLWHIV/AIDS and their families; emphasis on education interventions for men who have sex with men	Bronx, Brooklyn, Queens, Staten Island
HIV Law Project	Client advocacy	PLWHIV/AIDS	Bronx, Manhattan
Housing Works	Housing, health care, advocacy, job training	Homeless PLWHIV/AIDS	Citywide
Latino Commission on AIDS (LCOA)	Treatment education	Spanish-language dominant PLWHIV/AIDS and their service providers	Citywide
Life Force, Women Fighting AIDS	Education, advocacy, services	Women and families	Brooklyn

Organization	Service	Population	Area
Lower East Side Harm Reduction Center	Harm reduction	Injecting drug users	Lower East Side
Minority Task Force on AIDS (MTFA)	Client advocacy, services, referrals	Individuals and community-based service providers	Citywide
Momentum Project	Food and nutrition	PLWHIV/AIDS	Bronx, Brooklyn, Manhattan, Queens
Mothers' Voices (MV)	HIV prevention education	Parents	Citywide
New York AIDS Network (The Network)	Information exchange	N/A	Citywide
New York Harm Reduction Educators	Case management, harm reduction	PLWHIV/AIDS, people at high risk	Manhattan, Bronx
People With AIDS Health Group (PWA HG)	Buyer's club	PLWHIV/AIDS	Citywide
People with AIDS Coalition of New York (PWAC)	Information, outreach, and support programs	PLWHIV/AIDS	Citywide
Positive Health Project (PHP)	Support, education, syringe exchange	PLWHIV/AIDS	Citywide
St. Ann's Corner of Harm Reduction (SACHR)	Harm reduction	Injecting drug users	Bronx
Treatment Action Group (TAG)	Research advocacy	N/A	
Women and AIDS Resource Network (WARN)	Information dissemination	Women	Citywide

References

Abdul-Quader, A., D. Des Jarlais, A. Chatterjee, E. Hirky, and S. Friedman. 1999. "Interventions for Injecting Drug Users." In *Preventing HIV in Developing Countries: Biomedical And Behavioral Approaches*, ed. L. Gibney, R. J. DiClemente, and S. H. Vermund. New York: Plenum.

Abrahamson, Mark. 2004. *Global Cities*. New York: Oxford University Press.

Abu-Lughod, Janet. 1994. *From Urban Village to East Village: The Battle for New York's Lower East Side*. Oxford, UK: Blackwell, 1994.

ACLU. 1993. "Comments of the American Civil Liberties Union to the United States Sentencing Commission Regarding Disparity in Penalty between Crack and Powder Cocaine." October 26, 1993.

ACT UP. 1988. "The Working Document." New York: AIDS Coalition to Unleash Power.

ACT UP Women's Handbook Group. 1990. *Women, AIDS, and Activism*. Boston: South End Press.

Adam, Barry D. 1997. "Mobilizing around AIDS: Sites of Struggle in the Formation of AIDS Subjects." In *In Changing Times: Gay Men and Lesbians Encounter HIV/AIDS*, ed. M. Levine, P. Nardi, and J. Gagnon. Chicago: University of Chicago Press.

Ades, Paul. 1989. "The Unconstitutionality of 'Antihomeless' Laws: Ordinances Prohibiting Sleeping in Outdoor Public Areas as a Violation of the Right to Travel." *California Law Review* 77:595–627.

Aggleton, Peter. 1997. "Behavior Change Communication Strategies." *AIDS Education and Prevention* 9 (2): 111–23.

Allen, S., V. Mor, J. Fleishman, and J. Piette. 1995. "The Organizational Transformation of Advocacy: Community Based Organizations." *AIDS and Public Policy Journal* 10:48–59.

Altman, Dennis. 1988. "Legitimation through Disaster: AIDS and the Gay Movement." In *AIDS: The Burdens of History*, ed. Elizabeth Fee and Daniel M. Fox. Berkeley: University of California Press.

———. 1994. *Power and Community: Organizational and Cultural Responses to AIDS*. London: Taylor & Francis.

Alvarez, Sonia. 1998. "Latin American Feminists 'Go Global': Trends of the 1990s and Challenges for the New Millennium." In *Cultures of Politics, Politics of Cultures: Re-visioning Latin American Social Movements*, ed. Sonia Alvarez, Evelina Dagnino, and Arturo Escobar, 293–324. Boulder, CO: Westview Press.

Aminzade, Ronald. 1995. "Between Movement and Party: The Transformation of Mid-Nineteenth Century French Republicanism." In *The Politics of Social Protest: Comparative Perspectives on States and Social Movements*, ed. J. Craig Jenkins and Bert Klandermans, 39–62. Minneapolis: University of Minnesota Press.

Anastos, Kathryn, and Carola Marte. 1991 [1989]. "Women—the Missing Persons in the AIDS Epidemic." In *The AIDS Reader: Social, Political, and Ethical Issues*, ed. Nancy McKenzie. New York: Penguin Books.

Anderson, Benedict. 1991. *Imagined Communities: Reflections on the Origins and Spread of Nationalism*. London: Verso.

Anderson, W. 1991. "The New York Needle Trial: The Politics of Public Health in the Age of AIDS." *American Journal of Public Health* 81 (11): 1506–17.

Anglin, Mary. 1997. "Working from the Inside Out: Implications of Breast Cancer Activism for Biomedical Policies and Practices." *Social Science and Medicine* 44:1403–15.

Anslinger, Harry, and Will Oursler. 1961. *The Murderers: The Story of the Narcotic Gangs*. New York: Farrar, Strauss & Cudahy.

Aran, Ron, and David Rogers. 1990. "AIDS in the United States: Patient Care and Politics." In *Living with AIDS*, ed. Stephen R. Graubard. Cambridge, MA: MIT Press.

Arno, Peter S. 1986. "The Nonprofit Sector's Response to the AIDS Epidemic: Community-Based Services in San Francisco." *American Journal of Public Health* 76:1325-30.

Arno, Peter S., and Karyn Feiden. 1992. *Against the Odds: The Story of AIDS Drug Development*. New York: HarperCollins.

Backstrom, Charles, and Leonard Robins. 1995. "State AIDS Policy Making: Perspectives of Legislative Health Committee Chairs." *AIDS and Public Policy* 10 (4): 238–48.

Baldor, Lolita C. 2006. "Pentagon Lists Homosexuality as Disorder." *Associated Press*. June 20.

Baum, Joel. 1995. "The Changing Basis of Competition in Organizational Populations: The Manhattan Hotel Industry, 1898–1900." *Social Forces* 74 (1): 177–205.

Bayer, Ron, and Donald L. Kirp. 1992. "The United States: At the Center of the Storm." In *AIDS in the Industrialized Democracies: Passions, Politics, and Policies*, ed. David L. Kirp and Ronald Bayer. New Brunswick, NJ: Rutgers University Press.

Bearman, Peter S., and Kevin D. Everett. 1993. "The Structure of Social Protest, 1961–1983." *Social Networks* 15:171–200.

Benford, Robert. 1993. "Frame Disputes within the Nuclear Disarmament Movement." *Social Forces* 71:677–701.

Berer, Marge. 1993. *Women and HIV/AIDS: An International Resource Book; information, Action, and Resources on Women and HIV/AIDS, Reproductive Health, and Sexual Relationships.* London: Pandora.

Berry, Jeffrey M., and David F. Arons. 2003. *A Voice for Nonprofits.* Washington, DC: Brookings Institute.

Bielefeld, Wolfgang, and Richard Scotch. 1996. "Institutionalizing AIDS: Policy, Institutional Culture, and the Response to the HIV Epidemic in Dallas." *Research in Social Policy* 4:39–53.

Blau, Judith, and Gordana Rabenovic. 1991. "Interorganizational Relations of Nonprofit Organizations: An Exploratory Study." *Sociological Forum* 6 (2): 327–47.

Blendon, Robert J., and Karen Donelan. 1990. "AIDS and Discrimination: Public and Professional Perspectives." In *AIDS and the Health Care System*, ed. Lawrence O. Gostin. New Haven, CT: Yale University Press.

Bluthenthal, Ricky, Alex H. Kral, Elizabeth A. Erringer, and Brian R. Edlin. 1999. "Drug Paraphernalia Laws and Injection-Related Infectious Disease Risk among Drug Injectors." *Journal of Drug Issues* 29 (1): 1–16.

Booth, Karen M. 2000. "'Just Testing': Race, Sex, and the Media in New York's 'Baby AIDS' Debate." *Gender and Society* 14 (5): 644–61.

Bordt, Rebecca L. 1997. "How Alternative Ideas Become Institutions: The Case of Feminist Collectives." *Nonprofit and Voluntary Sector Quarterly* 26 (2): 132–55.

Borgatti, S. P., and M. G. Everett. 1992. "Notions of Position in Social Network Analysis." In *Sociological Methodology*, ed. P. Marsden. London: Basil Blackwell.

Bourdieu, Pierre. 1990. *The Logic of Practice.* Translated by Richard Nice. Stanford, CA: Stanford University Press.

Brown, Chip. 1992. "A Last Good Place to Live: Inside a Residence for the Homeless with AIDS." *Harper's Magazine.* February.

Brown, Michael P. 1997. *Replacing Citizenship: AIDS Activism and Radical Democracy.* New York: Guilford Press.

Buechler, Steven M. 1990. *Women's Movements in the United States: Woman Suffrage, Equal Rights, and Beyond.* New Brunswick, NJ: Rutgers University Press.

Buning, E., G. van Brussel, and G. van Santen. 1992. "The Impact of Harm Reduction Drug Policy on AIDS Prevention in Amsterdam." In *The Reduction of Drug-Related Harm*, ed. P. A. O'Hare, R. Newcombe, A. Mathews, E. C. Buning, and E. Drucker. London: Routledge.

Bureau of AIDS Epidemiology. 2005. "New York State HIV/AIDS Surveillance Semiannual Report, for Cases Diagnosed through December 2001." New York State Department of Health.

Bureau of HIV/AIDS Epidemiology. 1999. "AIDS Surveillance Quarterly Update: For Cases Reported through September 1999." New York State Department of Health.

Bureau of Ryan White CARE Services. 1995. "Title 1 Ryan White Comprehensive AIDS Resources Emergency (CARE) Relief Grant Program: Service Directory." New York: New York State Department of Health.

Burris, S., D. Finucane, H. Gallagher, and J. Grace. 1996. "The Legal Strategies Used in Operating Syringe Exchange Programs in the United States." *American Journal of Public Health* 86 (8): 1161–66.

Burstein, Paul. 1991. "Policy Domains: Organization, Culture and Policy Outcomes." *Annual Review of Sociology* 17:327–50.

Burt, Ronald S. 1992. *Structural Holes: The Social Structure of Competition*. Cambridge, MA: Harvard University Press.

Cain, Roy. 1995. "Community-Based AIDS Organizations and the State: Dilemmas of Dependence." *AIDS and Public Policy Journal* 10:83–93.

Caniglia, Beth Scaefer. 2001. "Informal Alliances vs. Institutional Ties: The Effects of Elite Alliances on Environmental TSMO Networks." *Mobilization* 6 (1): 37–54.

Case, Patricia, Thera Meehan, and T. Stephen Jones. 1998. "Arrests and Incarceration of Injecting Drug Users for Syringe Possession in Massachusetts: Implications for HIV Prevention." *Journal of Acquired Immune Deficiency Syndrome and Human Retrovirology* 18 (Suppl. 1): S71–S75.

Castells, Manuel. 1999 [2002]. "The Culture of Cities in the Information Age." In *The Castells Reader on Cities and Social Theory*, ed. Ida Susser, 369–89. Oxford: Blackwell.

Centers for Disease Control (CDC). 1981a. "*Pneumocystis* Pneumonia—Los Angeles." *Morbidity and Mortality Weekly Report* 30:250.

———. 1981b. "Kaposi's Sarcoma and *Pneumocystis* Pneumonia among Homosexual Men—New York City and California." *Morbidity and Mortality Weekly Report* 30:305–8.

———. 1982. Opportunistic Infections and Kaposi's Sarcoma among Haitians in the United States." *Morbidity and Mortality Weekly Report* 31:353–61.

———. 1983a. "An Evaluation of the Acquired Immunodeficiency Syndrome (AIDS) Reported in Health-Care Personnel—United States." *Morbidity and Mortality Weekly Report* 32:358–60.

———. 1983b. "Update: Acquired Immunodeficiency Syndrome (AIDS)—United States." *Morbidity and Mortality Weekly Report* 32:465–67.

———. 2000. *HIV/AIDS Surveillance Report*. December.

Center for Women Policy Studies. 1996. "Women and the CARE Act—Findings and Recommendations from a Process Evaluation of the Ryan White CARE Act Title I Planning Process." Washington, DC: Center for Women Policy Studies.

Chambré, Susan. n.d. "Voluntarism in the HIV Epidemic: Raising Resources for Community-Based Organizations in New York City and Sullivan County." Working Paper Series. The Aspen Institute.

———. 1996. "Uncertainty, Diversity, and Change: The AIDS Community in New York City." *Research in Community Sociology* 6:149–90.

———. 1997. "Civil Society, Differential Resources, and Organizational Development: HIV/AIDS Organizations in New York City, 1982–1992." *Nonprofit and Voluntary Sector Quarterly* 26:466–88.

Clifford, George. 1992. *The AIDS Epidemic in New York City: The Responses of Community Based Organizations, Political Action Groups, and Government from 1981 to 1990*. PhD diss., State University of New York at Albany.

Cohen, Cathy Jean. 1999. *The Boundaries of Blackness: AIDS and the Breakdown of Black Politics*. Chicago: University of Chicago Press.

Coleman, James. 1988. "Social Capital in the Creation of Human Capital." *American Journal of Sociology* 94:S94.

Courtwright, David, Herman Joseph, and Don Des Jarlais. 1989. *Addicts Who Survived: An Oral History of Narcotic Use in America*. Knoxville: University of Tennessee Press.

Couto, Richard A. 1993. "Narrative, Free Space, and Political Leadership in Social Movements." *The Journal of Politics* 55 (1): 57–79.

Crimp, Douglas, ed. 1992. "Right On, Girlfriend!" *Social Text* 33:2–18.

Crystal, Stephen, and Nina Glick Schiller. 1993. "Stigma and Homecoming: Family Caregiving and the 'Disaffiliated' Intravenous Drug User." In *The Social and Behavioral Aspects of AIDS: Advances in Medical Sociology*, ed. G. Albrecht and R. Zimmerman, vol. 3. Greenwich CT: JAI Press.

Curran, James W. 1986. "Acquired Immunodeficiency Syndrome: The Beginning, the Present, and the Future." In *AIDS, From the Beginning*, ed. Helene Cole and George Lundberg, xxi–xxvii. Chicago: American Medical Association.

Curtis, Russel, Jr., and Louis Zurcher Jr. 1975. "Multiple Resources of Protest Movements: The Multi-Organizational Field." *Social Forces* 52:53–61.

Cuthbert, Melinda. 1990. *Organizational Response to AIDS: The Politics of Policy-Setting*. PhD diss., Yale University, New Haven, CT.

Dalton, Harlon L. 1989. "AIDS in Blackface." *Daedalus* 118 (3): 205–27.

Deakin, Nicholas. 1995. "The Perils of Partnership: The Voluntary Sector and the State, 1945–1992." In *An Introduction to the Voluntary Sector*, ed. Justin Davis Smith, Colin Rochester, and Rodney Hedley. London: Routledge.

Della Porta, Donatella. 1988. "Recruitment Processes in Clandestine Political Organizations: Italian Left-Wing Terrorism." In *International Social Movement Research*. Greenwich, CT: JAI Press.

D'Eramo, John. 1987. "Ain't No Mountain High Enough." In *International Conferences on AIDS*, ed. J. C. Gluckman and E. Vilmer, 257–60, notes. Paris: Elsevier.

Des Jarlais, D., J. Guydish, S. Friedman, and H. Hagen. 2000. "HIV Prevention for Drug Users in Natural Settings." In *Handbook of HIV Prevention*, ed. John L. Peterson and Ralph J. DiClemente, 159–78. New York: Kluwer Academic/Plenum Publishers.

Diani, Mario. 2001. "Social Capital as Social Movement Outcome." In *Beyond Tocqueville: Civil Society and the Social Capital Debate in Comparative Perspective*, ed. Bob Edwards, Michael W. Foley, and Mario Diani, 207–18. Hanover, NH: Tufts.

Diaz, Rafael Miguel. 1997. "Latino Gay Men and Psycho-Cultural Barriers to AIDS Prevention." In *In Changing Times: Gay Men and Lesbians Encounter HIV/AIDS*, ed. M. Levine, P. Nardi, and J. Gagnon. Chicago: University of Chicago Press.

Dill, Ann. 1994. "Institutional Environments and Organizational Responses to AIDS." *Journal of Health and Social Behavior* 35:349–69.

DiMaggio, Paul. 1991. "Constructing an Organizational Field as a Professional Project: U.S. Art Museums, 1920–1940." In *The New Institutionalism in Organizational Analysis*, ed. Paul DiMaggio and Walter W. Powell. Chicago: University of Chicago Press.

DiMaggio, Paul, and Walter W. Powell. 1983. "The Iron Cage Revisited: Institutional Isomorphism and Collective Rationality in Organizational Fields." *American Sociological Review* 48:147–60.

———, ed. 1991. Introduction to *The New Institutionalism in Organizational Analysis*. Chicago: University of Chicago Press.

Doka, Kenneth J. 1997. *AIDS, Fear, and Society: Challenging the Dreaded Disease*. Washington, DC: Taylor & Francis.

Donovan, Mark C. 1997. "The Problem with Making AIDS Comfortable: Federal Policy Making and the Rhetoric of Innocence." *Journal of Homosexuality* 32 (3–4): 115–44.

Dunne, Richard. 1987. "New York City: Gay Men's Health Crisis." *AIDS: Public Policy Dimensions*, ed. John H. Griggs. New York: United Hospital Fund of New York.

Durkheim, Emile. 1964 [1933]. *The Division of Labor in Society*. New York: Free Press.

Duster, Troy. 1970. *The Legislation of Morality: Law, Drugs and Moral Judgement*. New York: The Free Press.

———. 1997. "Pattern, Purpose, and Race in the Drug War: The Crisis of Credibility in Criminal Justice." In *Crack in America: Demon Drugs and Social Justice*, ed. Craig Reinarman and Harry G. Levine, 260–87. Berkeley: University of California Press.

Eckholdt, H., J. Chin, J. Manzon-Santos, and D. Kim. 1997. "The Needs of Asians and Pacific Islanders Living with HIV in New York City." *AIDS Education and Prevention* 9:493–504.

Edwards, Bob. 1994. "Semiformal Organizational Structure among Social Movement Organizations: An Analysis of the U.S. Peace Movement." *Nonprofit and Voluntary Sector Quarterly* 23:309–33.

Edwards, Bob, Michael W. Foley, and Mario Diani, eds. 2001. *Beyond Tocqueville: Civil Society and the Social Capital Debate in Comparative Perspective*. Hanover, NH: University Press of New England.

Elbaz, Gilbert. 1992. *The Sociology of AIDS Activism: The Case of ACT UP/New York, 1987–1992*. PhD diss., City University of New York.

Elovich, Richard, and Rod Sorge. 1991. "Toward a Community-Based Needle Exchange for New York City." *AIDS & Public Policy Journal* 6 (4): 165–72.

Epstein, Stephen. 1996. *Impure Science: AIDS, Activism, and the Politics of Knowledge*. Berkeley: University of California Press.

Escobar, Arturo. 2004. "Beyond the Third World: Imperial Globality, Global Coloniality, and Anti-globalisation Social Movements." *Third World Quarterly* 25 (1): 207–20.

Evans, Peter. 1997. "The Eclipse of the State? Reflections on Stateness in an Era of Globalization." *World Politics* 50 (1): 62–87.

Farmer, Paul. 1992. *AIDS and Accusation: Haiti and the Geography of Blame*. Berkeley: University of California Press.

Fee, Elizabeth, and Daniel M. Fox, eds. 1988. *AIDS: The Burdens of History*. Berkeley: University of California Press.

Finkelstein, Ruth, and Amanda Vogel. 1999. *Towards a Comprehensive Plan for Syringe Exchange in New York City*. New York: New York Academy of Medicine.

Fleishman, J., V. Mor, J. Piette, and S. Allen. 1992. "Organizing AIDS Service Consortia: Lead Agency Identity and Consortium Cohesion." *Social Service Review* (December 1992): 547–70.

Freeman, Jo. 1975. *The Politics of Women's Liberation: A Case Study of an Emerging Social Movement and Its Relation to the Policy Process.* New York: David McKay Company.

Freudenberg, Nicholas. 1990. "AIDS Prevention in the United States: Lessons from the First Decade." *International Journal of Health Services* 20:589–99.

Friedman, Samuel, and Yolanda Serrano. 1989. "AIDS-Related Organizing of IV Drug Users from the Outside." *The Newsletter of the International Working Group on AIDS and IV Drug Use* 4 (2): 2–4.

Galatowitch, Paul. 1996. *An Organizational, Institutional and Cultural Analysis of New Haven, Connecticut's Response to the AIDS Epidemic.* PhD diss., Yale University, New Haven, CT.

———. 1999. "The Failure of Success: Institutional Isomorphism and Organizational Responses to AIDS." Paper presented at the 94th annual meeting of the American Sociological Association, Chicago, IL, August 6–10.

Gamson, Joshua. 1995. "Must Identity Movements Self-Destruct? A Queer Dilemma." *Social Problems* 42:101–18.

Gerlach, Luther, and Virginia Hine. 1970. *People, Power, Change: Movements of Social Transformation.* Indianapolis: Bobbs-Merrill.

Glick Schiller, Nina. 2002. "What's Wrong with This Picture? The Hegemonic Construction of Culture in AIDS Research in the United States." *Medical Anthropology Quarterly* 6 (3): 237–54.

Gottman, J. 1989. "What Are Cities Becoming the Center Of?" In *Cities in a Global Society*, ed. R. Knight and G. Gappart. Newbury Park, CA: Sage.

Gould, Roger. 1991. " Multiple Networks and Mobilization in the Paris Commune, 1971." *American Sociological Review* 56:716–29.

Granovetter, Mark. 1985. "Economic Action and Social Structure: The Problem of Embeddedness." *American Journal of Sociology* 91 (3): 481–510.

Gray, Mike. 2000. *Drug Crazy: How We Got into This Mess and How We Can Get Out.* New York: Routledge.

Greenstone, J. David, and Paul E. Peterson. 1973. *Race and Authority in Urban Politics: Community Participation and the War on Poverty.* New York: Russell Sage Foundation.

Guo, Chao, and Muhittin Acar. 2005. "Understanding Collaboration among Nonprofit Organizations: Combining Resource Dependency, Institutional, and Network Perspectives." *Nonprofit and Voluntary Sector Quarterly* 34 (3): 340–61.

Gupta, Akhil, and James Ferguson. 1991. "Beyond 'Culture': Space, Identity, and the Politics of Difference." *Cultural Anthropology* 7 (1): 6–23.

Gusfield, Joseph. 1981. *The Culture of Public Problems.* Chicago: University of Chicago Press.

Haines, Herbert H. 1984. "Black Radicalism and the Funding of Civil Rights: 1957–1970." *Social Problems* 32:31–43.

Hall, Stuart. 1990. "Cultural Identity and Diaspora." In *Identity: Community, Culture, Difference*, ed. Jonathan Rutherford. London: Lawrence & Wishart.

Hallett, Michael A., and David Cannella. 1994. "Gatekeeping through Media Format: Strategies of Voice for the HIV-Positive via Human Interest News Formats and Organizations." *Journal of Homosexuality* 26 (4): 111–34.

Harrington, Mark. 1994. "The Community Research Initiative (CRI) of New York: Clinical Research and Prevention Treatments." In *AIDS Prevention and Services: Community Based Research*, ed. Johannes P. Van Vugt. Westport, CT: Bergin & Garvey.

———. 1998. "From Acting Up to Acts of Congress, AIDS Activist Reviews and Critiques a Decade of Social Change." *TAGLine* 5 (9). Treatment Action Group.

Hathaway, Will, and David S. Meyer. 1994. "Competition and Cooperation in Social Movement Coalitions: Lobbying for Peace in the 1980s." *Berkeley Journal of Sociology* 38:156–83.

Hay, Louise. 1984. *You Can Heal Your Life*. Santa Monica, CA: Hay House.

Healey, K. M. 1988. "State and Local Experience with Drug Paraphernalia Laws." Washington, DC: National Institute of Justice.

Heckathorn, Douglas D., Robert S. Broadhead, Denise L. Anthony, and David L. Weakliem. 1999. "AIDS and Social Networks: HIV Prevention through Network Mobilization." *Sociological Focus* 32 (2): 159–79.

Henman, A., D. Paone, D. Des Jarlais, L. Kochems, and S. Friedman. 1998. "Injection Drug Users as Social Actors: A Stigmatized Community's Participation in the Syringe Exchange Programmes of New York City." *AIDS Care* 10 (4): 397–408.

Hispanic AIDS Forum. n.d. "History and Mission." Pamphlet.

Hodson, Randy. 1998. "Organizational Ethnographies: An Underutilized Resource in the Sociology of Work." *Social Forces* 76 (4): 1173–1208.

Hoek, J. A. R. van den, H. J. A. van Haastrecht, and R. A. Coutinho. 1989. "Risk Reduction among Intravenous Drug Users in Amsterdam under the Influence of AIDS." *American Journal of Public Health* 79:1355–57.

HRA. 2000. "HRA Facts." New York City: Human Resources Agency.

HRSA. 2002. "CARE Act Overview and Funding." U. S. Department of Health and Human Services, Health Resources and Services Administration, HIV/AIDS Bureau.

———. 2004. "Ryan White CARE Act: Before the CARE Act; 1985–90." Health Resources and Services Administration, HIV/AIDS Bureau.

Iritani, Evelyn. 2005. "From the Streets to the Inner Sanctum." *Los Angeles Times*, February 20, 2005.

James, Estelle. 1987. "The Nonprofit Sector in Comparative Perspective." *The Nonprofit Sector: A Research Handbook*, ed. W. W. Powell, 43–54. New Haven, CT: Yale University Press.

Jasper, James. 1997. *The Art of Moral Protest: Culture, Biography, and Creativity in Social Movements*. Chicago: University of Chicago Press.

Jenkins, J. C., and Craig M. Eckert. 1986. "Channeling Black Insurgency: Elite Patronage and Professional Social Movement Organizations in the Development of the Black Movement." *American Sociological Review* 51:812–29.

Jensen, Eric, and Jurg Gerber. 1998. "The Social Construction of Drug Problems: An Historical Overview." In *The New War on Drugs: Symbolic Politics and Criminal Justice Policy*, ed. Eric L. Jensen and Jurg Gerber, 1–23. Highland Heights, KY: Academy of Criminal Justice Sciences/Anderson Publishing Company.

Jepperson, Ronald L. 1991. "Institutions, Institutional Effects, and Institutionalism." In *The New Institutionalism in Organizational Analysis*, ed. Walter W. Powell and Paul J. DiMaggio, 143–63. Chicago: University of Chicago Press.

Joseph, Stephen C. 1992. *Dragon within the Gates: The Once and Future AIDS Epidemic*. New York: Carroll & Graf Publishers.

Joseph, Stephen, and Don Des Jarlais. 1989. "Needle and Syringe Exchange as a Method of AIDS Epidemic Control." *AIDS Updates* 2:1–8.

Joslin, Daphne, ed. 2002. *Invisible Caregivers: Older Adults Raising Children in the Wake of HIV/AIDS*. New York: Columbia University Press.

Kayal, Philip. 1993. *Bearing Witness: Gay Men's Health Crisis and the Politics of AIDS*. Boulder, CO: Westview Press.

Kelley, Margaret, Howard Lune, and Sheigla Murphy. 2005. "Doing Syringe Exchange: Organizational Transformation and Volunteer Commitment." *Nonprofit and Voluntary Sector Quarterly* 34 (3): 362–86.

Kelly, J. A., and St. Lawrence, J. S. 1990. "The Impact of Community-Based Groups to Help Persons Reduce HIV Infection Risk Behaviors." *AIDS Care* 2 (1): 25–35.

Kinsella, James. 1989. *Covering the Plague: AIDS and the American Media*. New Brunswick, NJ: Rutgers University Press.

Kirp, David L. 1989. *Learning by Heart: AIDS and Schoolchildren in America's Communities*. New Brunswick, NJ: Rutgers University Press.

Kirp, David L., and Ronald Bayer. 1992. *AIDS in the Industrialized Democracies: Passions, Politics, and Policies*. New Brunswick, NJ: Rutgers University Press.

——. 1993. "The Politics." In *Dimensions of AIDS Prevention: Needle Exchange*, ed. Jeff Stryker and Mark D. Smith. Menlo Park, CA: The Henry J. Kaiser Family Foundation.

Klandermans, Bert. 1992. "The Social Construction of Protest and Mulitorganizational Fields." In *Frontiers of Social Movement Theory*, ed. A. Morris and C. Mueller. New Haven, CT: Yale University Press.

——. 1993. "A Theoretical Framework for Comparisons of Social Movement Participation." *Sociological Forum* 8 (3): 383–402.

Kleidman, Robert. 1994. "Volunteer Activism and Professionalism in Social Movement Organizations." *Social Problems* 41:257–76.

Klein, Naomi. 2002. "The Vision Thing: Were the DC and Seattle Protests Unfocused, or Are Critics Missing the Point?" *From ACT UP to the WTO: Urban Protest and Community Building in the Era of Globalization*, ed. Benjamin Shepard and Ronald Hayduk, 264–73. New York: Verso.

Kochems, Lee M., Denise Paone, Don C. Des Jarlais, Immanuel Ness, Jessica Clark, and Samuel R. Friedman. 1996. "The Transition for Underground to Legal Syringe Exchange: The New York City Experience." *AIDS Education and Prevention* 8 (6): 471–89.

Koester, Stephen K. 1994. "Copping, Running, and Paraphernalia Laws: Contextual Variables and Needle Risk Behavior among Injecting Drug Users in Denver." *Human Organization* 53 (3): 287–95.

Kohn, Melvin. 1993. "Doing Social Research under Conditions of Radical Social Change: The Biography of an Ongoing Research Project." *Social Psychology Quarterly* 56 (1): 4–20.

Kowalewski, Mark R. 1988. "Double Stigma and Boundary Maintenance." *Journal of Contemporary Ethnography* 17 (2): 211–28.

Kramer, Larry. 1983. "1,112 and Counting." *The New York Native* 59 (March): 14–27.

———. 1989. *Reports from the Holocaust: The Making of an Activist*. New York: St. Martin's Press.

Lemelle, Anthony, and Charlene Harrington. 1998. "The Political Economy of Caregiving for People with HIV/AIDS." In *The Political Economy of AIDS*, ed. Merrill Singer, 149–66. Amityville, NY: Baywood Publishing Company.

Leonhardt, F. 1980. *Banning Drug Paraphernalia*. Salem, OR: Legislative Research.

Lichterman, Paul. 1995. "Piecing Together Multicultural Community: Cultural Differences in Community Building among Grass-roots Environmentalists." *Social Problems* 42:513.

Lin, Nan. 2001. *Social Capital: A Theory of Social Structure and Action*. New York: Cambridge University Press.

Lune, Howard. 2002a. "Weathering the Storm: Nonprofit Organization Survival Strategies in a Hostile Climate." *Nonprofit and Voluntary Sector Quarterly* 31 (4): 463–83.

———. 2002b. "Reclamation Activism in Anti-drug Organizing in the U.S." *Social Movement Studies* 1 (2): 147–68.

Lune, Howard, and Miranda Martinez. 1999. "Old Structures, New Relations: How Community Development Credit Unions Define Organizational Boundaries." *Sociological Forum* 14 (4): 609–34.

Lune, Howard, and Hillary Oberstein. 2001. "Embedded Systems: The Case of HIV/AIDS Nonprofit Organizations in New York City." *Voluntas* 12 (1): 17–33.

MacKinnon, Kenneth. 1992. *The Politics of Popular Representation: Reagan, Thatcher, AIDS, and the Movies*. Rutherford: Farleigh Dickinson University Press.

MacNair, Ray, Leigh Fowler, and John Harris. 2000. "The Diversity Functions of Organizations That Confront Oppression: The Evolution of Three Social Movements." *Journal of Community Practice* 7 (2): 71–88.

Malinowsky, H. Robert, and Gerald J. Perry, eds. 1991. *AIDS Information Sourcebook*. 3rd ed. Phoenix: Oryx Press.

Mansbridge, Jane J. 1986. *Why We Lost the ERA*. Chicago: University of Chicago Press.

———. 1993. In *Democratic Community*, ed. John W. Chapman and Ian Shapiro, 339–95. New York: New York University Press.

McAdam, Doug. 1982. *Political Process and the Development of Black Insurgency, 1930–1970*. Chicago: University of Chicago Press.

———. 1988. "Micromobilization Contexts and Recruitment to Activism." *International Social Movement Research* 1:12554.

McCarthy, John, David Britt, and Mark Wolfson. 1991. "The Institutional Channeling of Social Movements by the State in the United States." *Research in Social Movements, Conflict and Change* 13:45–76.

McCarthy, John D., and Mayer Zald. 1977. "Mobilization and Social Movements: A Partial Theory." *American Journal of Sociology* 82:1212–41.

McDermott, Peter. 1992. "New York through the Eye of a Needle." *The Face Magazine*, October.

McKinney, Martha M. 1993. "Consortium Approaches to the Delivery of HIV Services under the Ryan White CARE Act." *AIDS & Public Policy Journal* 8:115–25.

McPherson, J. Miller. 1982. "Hypernetwork Sampling: Duality and Differentiation among Voluntary Organizations." *Social Networks* 3:225–49.

MDHG, Interest Group for Drug Users. 1992. *Drugs and AIDS in the Netherlands— the Interests of Drug Users*. Amsterdam: MDHG.

Merton, Vanessa. 1990. "Community-Based AIDS Research." *Evaluation Review* 14:502–37.

Meyer, David S., and Suzanne Staggenborg. 1998. "Countermovement Dynamics in Federal Systems: A Comparison of Abortion Politics in Canada and the United States." *Research in Political Sociology* 8:209–40.

Meyer, David S., and Nancy Whittier. 1994. "Social Movement Spillover." *Social Problems* 41:277–97.

Michels, Robert. [1935] 1968. *Political Parties: A Sociological Study of the Oligarchical Tendencies of Modern Democracy*. Translated by Eden Paul and Cedar Paul. New York: Free Press.

Milofsky, Carl. 1988. "Scarcity and Community: A Resource Allocation Theory of Community and Mass Society Organizations." In *Community Organizations: Studies in Resource Mobilization and Exchange*, ed. C. Milofsky, 16–41. New York: Oxford University Press.

Minkoff, Debra. 1994. "From Service Provision to Institutional Advocacy: The Shifting Legitimacy of Organizational Forms." *Social Forces* 72 (4): 943–69.

Mor, V., J. Fleishman, S. Allen, and J. Piette. 1994. *Networking AIDS Services*. Ann Arbor, MI: Health Administration Press.

Morgen, Sandra. 1986. "The Dynamics of Cooptation in a Feminist Health Clinic." *Social Science and Medicine* 23 (2): 201–10.

Morris, Aldon. 1984. *The Origin of the Civil Rights Movement: Black Communities Organizing for Change*. New York: Free Press.

———. 2000. "Reflections on Social Movement Theory: Criticisms and Proposals." *Contemporary Sociology* 29 (2): 445–54.

Moss, A. R. 2000. "Epidemiology and the Politics of Syringe Exchange." *American Journal of Public Health* 90 (9): 1385–87.

Moynihan, Daniel Patrick. 1969. *Maximum Feasible Misunderstanding*. New York: Free Press.

Musto, David F. 1999. *The American Disease: Origins of Narcotic Control*. Oxford: Oxford University Press.

National Commission on AIDS. 1993. *The Final Report of the National Commission on AIDS*. Washington, DC: Government Printing Office.

Navarre, Max. 1988. "Fighting the Victim Label." In *AIDS: Cultural Analysis/ Cultural Activism*, ed. Douglas Crimp. Cambridge, MA: MIT Press.

Needle, R., S. Coyle, J. Normand, E. Lambert, and H. Cesari. 1998. "HIV Prevention with Drug Using Populations—Current Status and Future Prospects: Introduction and Overview." *Public Health Reports* 113 (Suppl. 1), S4–S18.

New York City Department of Health. 1999. "New York City Ryan White Title I Service Directory." Bureau of Ryan White CARE Services.

New Yorker. 1992. "Battle Fatigue." November 9, 1992, 39–41.

Oliver, Christine. 1991. "Strategic Responses to Institutional Processes." *Academy of Management Review* 16 (1): 145–79.

ONDCP. 1999. *National Drug Control Strategy: 1999*. Washington, DC: Office of National Drug Control Policy.

Oppenheimer, Gerald M. 1988. "In the Eye of the Storm: The Epidemiological Construction of AIDS." In *AIDS: The Burdens of History*, ed. Elizabeth Fee and Daniel M. Fox, 267–300. Berkeley: University of California Press.

Padgug, Robert. 1987. "Gay Villain, Gay Hero: Homosexuality and the Social Construction of AIDS." In *Passion and Power: Sexuality in History*, ed. Kathy Peiss and Christina Simmons. Philadelphia: Temple University Press.

Pascal, Chris. 1988. "Intravenous Drug Abuse and AIDS Transmission: Federal and State Laws Regulating Needle Availability." In *Needle Sharing among Intravenous Drug Abusers: National and International Perspectives*, ed. R. J. Battles and R. W. Pickens. Washington, DC: National Institute on Drug Abuse, Monograph Series 80.

Patton, Cindy. 1990. *Inventing AIDS*. New York: Routledge.

Penner, Susan. 1995. "A Study of Coalitions among HIV/AIDS Service Organizations." *Sociological Perspectives* 38:217–39.

Perrow, C., and M. Guillèn. 1990. *The AIDS Disaster: The Failure of Organizations in New York and the Nation*. New Haven, CT: Yale University Press.

Peterson, John L. 1997. "AIDS-Related Risks and Same-Sex Behaviors among African American Men." *In Changing Times: Gay Men and Lesbians Encounter HIV/AIDS*, M. Levine, P. Nardi, and J. Gagnon. Chicago: University of Chicago Press.

Philips, Susan D. 1991. "Meaning and Structure in Social Movements: Mapping the Network of National Canadian Women's Organizations." *Canadian Journal of Political Science* 24:755–82.

Pizzorno, Alessandro. 1987. "Politics Unbound." In *Changing Boundaries of the Political: Essays on the Evolving Balance between the State and Society, Public and Private in Europe*, ed. Charles Maier, 27–62. Cambridge, MA: Cambridge University Press.

Portes, Alexandro. 1998. "Social Capital: Its Origins and Applications in Modern Sociology." *Annual Review of Sociology* 24:1–24.

Powell, Walter W. 1991. "Expanding the Scope of Institutional Analysis." In *The New Institutionalism in Organizational Dynamics*, ed. Paul DiMaggio and Walter W. Powell. Chicago: University of Chicago Press.

Poz Magazine. 1997. "True Colors." July.

Presidential Commission on HIV. 1992. *Report of the Presidential Commission on HIV*. Washington, DC: Government Printing Office.

Presidential Commission on the HIV Epidemic. 1988. *Report of the Presidential Commission on the Human Immunodeficiency Virus Epidemic*. Washington, DC: Government Printing Office.

Quam, Michael, and Nancy Ford. 1990. "AIDS Policies and Practices in the United States." In *Action on AIDS*, Barbara Misztal and David Moss. New York: Greenwood Press.

Quimby, Ernest. 1993. "Obstacles to Reducing AIDS among African Americans." *Journal of Black Psychology* 19:215–22.

Reinarman, Craig, and Harry Levine, eds. 1997. *Crack in America: Demon Drugs and Social Justice*. Berkeley: University of California Press.

Reinfeld, Rev. Margaret R. 1994. "The Gay Men's Health Crisis: A Model for Community Based Intervention." In *AIDS Prevention and Services: Community Based Research*, ed. Johannes P. Van Vugt. Westport, CT: Bergin & Garvey.

Rosenthal, Naomi, Meryl Fingrutd, Michele Ethier, Roberta Karant, and David McDonald. 1990. "Social Movements and Network Analysis: A Case Study of Nineteenth-Century Women's Reform in New York State." *American Journal of Sociology* 5:1022–54.

Russo, Vito. 1988. "Why We Fight." Video transcript of speech: ACT UP demonstration in Albany, NY, May 9, and the ACT UP demonstration at the Department of Health and Human Services, Washington, DC, October 10. www.actupny.org/documents/whfight.html (accessed April 2006).

Salamon, Lester, and Wojciech Sokolowski, eds. 2004. *Global Civil Society: Dimensions of the Nonprofit Sector*. Bloomfield, CT: Kumarian Press.

Sandalow, Marc. 2002. "Jesse Helms—Global AIDS Activist." *San Francisco Chronicle*, Monday, April 1, B7.

Sassen, Saskia. 1994. *Cities in a World Economy*. Thousand Oaks, CA: Pine Forge.

Schneider, Beth. 1997. "Owning an Epidemic: The Impact of AIDS on Small-City Lesbian and Gay Communities." In *In Changing Times: Gay Men and Lesbians Encounter HIV/AIDS*, ed. M. Levine, P. Nardi, and J. Gagnon, 145–70. Chicago: University of Chicago Press.

Seibel, Wolfgang. 1989. "The Function of Mellow Weakness: Nonprofit Organizations as Problem Nonsolvers in Germany." In *The Nonprofit Sector in International Perspective*, ed. Estelle James. Oxford: Oxford University Press.

Selznick, Philip. 1949. *TVA and the Grassroots*. Berkeley: University of California Press.

Sennett, Richard. 1992. *The Fall of Public Man*. New York: W. W. Norton & Company.

Shilts, R. 1987. *And the Band Played On: Politics, People, and the AIDS Epidemic*. New York: Penguin Books.

Shreve, Anita. 1989. *Women Together, Women Alone: The Legacy of the Consciousness Raising Movement*. New York: Viking.

Siegel, K. S., H. Lune, and I. Meyer. 1998. "Stigma Management among Gay/Bisexual Men with HIV/AIDS." *Qualitative Sociology* 21 (1).

Silverman, Mervyn. 1987. "San Francisco: Coordinated Community Response." In *AIDS: Public Policy Dimensions*, ed. John Griggs. New York: United Hospital Fund of New York.

Simon, Harry. 1982. "Towns without Pity: A Constitutional and Historical Analysis of Official Efforts to Drive Homeless Persons from American Cities." *Tulane Law Review* 66 (4): 631–76.

Smith, Steven Rathgeb, and Michael Lipsky. 1993. *Nonprofits for Hire: The Welfare State in the Age of Contracting*. Cambridge, MA: Harvard University Press.

Snow, David A., Louis A. Zurcher Jr., and Sheldon Ekland-Olson. 1980. "Social Networks and Social Movements: A Microstructural Approach to Differential Recruitment." *American Sociological Review* 45:787–801.

Sontag, Susan. 1989. "AIDS & Its Metaphors." In *Illness as Metaphor* and *AIDS & Its Metaphors*. New York: Anchor Books.

Spalter-Roth, Roberta, and Ronnee Schreiber. 1995. "Outsider Issues and Insider Tactics: Strategic Tensions in the Women's Policy Network During the 1980s." In *Feminist Organizations: Harvest of the New Women's Movement*, ed. Myra Marx Ferree and Patricia Yancey Martin. Philadelphia: Temple University Press.

Spencer, J. William. 1993. "Making 'Suitable Referrals': Social Workers' Construction and Use of Informal Referral Networks." *Sociological Perspectives* 36: 271–85.

Starhawk. 2002. "How We Really Shut down the WTO." In *From ACT UP to the WTO: Urban Protest and Community Building in the Era of Globalization*, Benjamin Shepard and Ronald Hayduk, 52–56. New York: Verso.

Stimson, G. V., L. J. Aldritt, K. A. Dolan, M. C. Donoghoe, and R. A. Lart. 1988. "Injecting Equipment Exchange Schemes: Final Report." Monitoring Research Group, Sociology Department, Goldsmith's College, London, 2–4.

Stoller, Nancy. 1995. "Lesbian Involvement in the AIDS Epidemic: Changing Roles and Generational Differences." In *Women Resisting AIDS: Feminist Strategies of Empowerment*, Beth Schneider and Nancy Stoller. Philadelphia: Temple University Press.

———. 1997. "From Feminism to Polymorphous Activism: Lesbians in AIDS Organizations." In *In Changing Times: Gay Men and Lesbians Encounter HIV/AIDS*, ed. Martin Levine, Peter Nardi, and John Gagnon. Chicago: University of Chicago Press.

———. 1998. *Lessons from the Damned: Queers, Whores, and Junkies Respond to AIDS*. New York: Routledge.

Stoneburner, Rand L., Mary Anne Chiasson, Isaac B. Weisfuse, and Pauline A. Thomas. 1990. "Editorial Review: The Epidemic of AIDS and HIV-1 Infection among Heterosexuals in New York City." *AIDS* 4:99–106.

Suttles, Gerald D. 1976. "Urban Ethnography: Situational and Normative Accounts." *Annual Review of Sociology* 2:1–18.

Tarrow, Sidney. 1994. *Power in Movement: Social Movements, Collective Action, and Politics*. Cambridge: Cambridge University Press.

Taylor, Verta. 1989. "Social Movement Continuity: The Women's Movement in Abeyance." *American Sociological Review* 54:761–75.

Taylor, Verta, and Nancy Whittier. 1995. "Analytic Approaches to Social Movement Culture: The Culture of the Women's Movement." In *Social Movements and Culture*, ed. H. Johnston and B. Klandermans. Minneapolis: University of Minnesota Press.

Thomas, Stephen B., and Sandra Crouse Quinn. 1991. "The Tuskegee Syphilis Study, 1932 to 1972: Implications for HIV Education and AIDS Risk Education Programs in the Black Community." *American Journal of Public Health* 81:1498–1504.

Tillett, D. 1982. "Banning the Head Shop: State Drug Paraphernalia Laws." In *CSG Backgrounder*, Lexington, KY: States Information Center. May.

Tilly, Charles. 1978. *From Mobilization to Revolution*. Reading, MA: Addison-Wesley.

———. 1996. "Contentious Repertoires in Great Britain." In *Repertoires and Cycles of Collective Action*, ed. Mark Traugott. Durham and London: Duke University Press.

Tocqueville, Alexis de. 1945 [1848]. *Democracy in America*. Vol. 1. New York: Vintage Books.

Tolbert, Pamela S., and Lynn G. Zucker. 1983. "Institutional Sources of Change in the Formal Structure of Organizations: The Diffusion of Civil Service Reform, 1880–1935." *Administrative Science Quarterly* 28:22–39.

Treichler, Paula A. 1988. "AIDS, Homophobia, and Biomedical Discourse: An Epidemic of Signification." In *AIDS: Cultural Analysis/Cultural Activism*, ed. Douglas Crimp. Cambridge, MA: MIT Press.

Turner, Ralph H., and Lewis M. Killian. 1957. *Collective Behavior*. Englewood Cliffs, NJ: Prentice-Hall Inc.

U.S. Department of Health and Human Services (DHHS). 1995. *HIV/AIDS Surveillance Report*. Vol. 7 (2). Atlanta: Department of Health and Human Services and the Centers for Disease Control and Prevention.

Useem, Michael, and Mayer Zald. 1982. "From Pressure Group to Social Movement: Organizational Dilemmas of the Effort to Promote Nuclear Power." *Social Problems* 30:144–56.

Van Vugt, Johannes. 1994. Introduction to *AIDS Prevention and Services: Community Based Research*, ed. Johannes Van Vugt. Westport, CT: Bergin & Garvey.

Vargas, Virginia. 2003. "Feminism, Globalization and the Global Justice and Solidarity Movement." *Cultural Studies* 17 (6): 905–20.

Wachter, Robert W. 1991. *The Fragile Coalition: Scientists, Activists, and AIDS*. New York: St. Martin's Press.

Wallace, Rodrick. 1992. "Public Policy and AIDS in New York City: The Legacy of 'Planned Shrinkage.'" *AIDS and Public Policy Journal* 7 (3): 153–57.

Watney, Simon. 1987. "The Spectacle of AIDS." In *AIDS: Cultural Analysis/Cultural Activism*, ed. Douglas Crimp. Cambridge, MA: MIT Press.

Weber, Max. 1978 [1922]. *Economy and Society: An Outline of Interpretive Sociology*, edited by G. Roth and C. Wittich. Berkeley: University of California Press.

Weisbrod, Burton A. 1988. *The Nonprofit Economy*. Cambridge, MA: Harvard University Press.

Weitz, Rose. 1991. *Life with AIDS*. New Brunswick, NJ: Rutgers University Press.

White, Harrison. 1992. *Identity and Control*. Princeton, NJ: Princeton University Press.

Whitman, C. T. 1998. "Governor Lauds U.S. Drug Czar's Opposition to Needle Exchange Programs." News release, April 21. State of New Jersey: Office of the Governor.

Wiewel, Wim, and Albert Hunter. 1985. "The Interorganizational Network as a Resource: A Comparative Case Study on Organizational Genesis." *Administrative Science Quarterly* 30:482–96.

Winkle, Curtis. 1991. "Inequality and Power in the Nonprofit Sector: A Comparative Analysis of AIDS—Related Services for Gay Men and Intravenous Drug Users in Chicago." *Nonprofit and Voluntary Sector Quarterly* 20.

Wolch, Jennifer. 1990. *The Shadow State: Government and Voluntary Sector in Transition*. New York: The Foundation Center.

Wolfe, Maxine. 1994. "The AIDS Coalition to Unleash Power (ACT UP): A Direct Model of Community Research for AIDS Prevention," in *AIDS Prevention and Services: Community Based Research*, Johannes P. Van Vugt. Westport, CT: Bergin & Garvey.

———. 1997. "After Ten Years: The Realities of the Crisis, Direct Action, and Setting the Agenda." Plenary session talk at the Conference on AIDS Activism, Hunter College. March.

Working Group on Social and Human Issues. 1991. *Report of the Working Group on Social and Human Issues to the National Commission on AIDS*. Washington, DC: Government Printing Office.

York, Alan, and Esther Zychlinski. 1996. "Competing Nonprofit Organizations also Collaborate." *Nonprofit Management and Leadership* 7:15–27.

Young, Iris Marion. 1990. "The Ideal of Community and the Politics of Difference." In *Feminism/Postmodernism*, ed. Linda Nicholson. New York: Routledge.

Zald, Mayer, and John D. McCarthy. 1987. "Appendix: The Trend of Social Movements in America: Professionalism and Resource Mobilization." In *Social Movements in an Organizational Society: Collected Essays*, ed. M. Zald and J. McCarthy, 337–91. New Brunswick: Transaction Books.

Index

About the Author

Howard Lune is assistant professor of sociology and the former director of the Urban Studies Program at William Paterson University of New Jersey. He studies formal and informal organizations, community mobilization efforts, nonprofit organizations, and transnational urban politics. Dr. Lune has also written about sociology's role in contemporary democratic states.